D0293967

NATURAL
WONDERFOODS

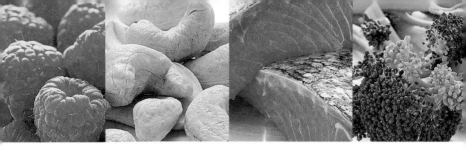

NATURAL
WONDERFOODS

100 AMAZING FOODS FOR
· HEALING · IMMUNE-BOOSTING ·
· FITNESS-ENHANCING · ANTI-AGEING ·

dbp

DUNCAN BAIRD PUBLISHERS
LONDON

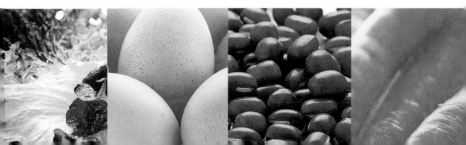

Natural Wonderfoods
Paula Bartimeus, Charlotte Haigh, Sarah Merson, Sarah Owen and Janet Wright

First published in the United Kingdom and Ireland in 2011 by
Duncan Baird Publishers Ltd
Sixth Floor, Castle House
75–76 Wells Street
London W1T 3QH

Conceived, created and designed by Duncan Baird Publishers

Copyright © Duncan Baird Publishers 2011
Text copyright © Paula Bartimeus 2009, 2011; Charlotte Haigh 2005, 2011; Sarah Owen 2009,
2011; Janet Wright 2008, 2011; Duncan Baird Publishers 2006, 2007, 2011
Commissioned photography copyright © Duncan Baird Publishers 2005, 2006, 2007, 2008,
2009, 2011

The right of Paula Bartimeus, Charlotte Haigh, Sarah Merson, Sarah Owen and
Janet Wright to be identified as the Authors of this text has been asserted in accordance
with the Copyright, Designs and Patents Act of 1988.

All rights reserved. No part of this book may be reproduced in any form or by any
electronic or mechanical means, including information storage and retrieval systems,
without permission in writing from the publisher, except by a reviewer who may quote
brief passages in a review.

Managing Editor: Grace Cheetham
Editor: Ingrid Court-Jones
Managing Designer: Manisha Patel
Designer: Rachel Cross
Photographs by: Simon Scott, Simon Smith and Toby Scott, and William Lingwood

British Library Cataloguing-in-Publication Data:
A CIP record for this book is available from the British Library

ISBN: 978-1-84483-929-2

10 9 8 7 6 5 4 3

Typeset in Warnock Pro
Colour reproduction by Colourscan, Singapore
Printed in Malaysia for Imago

Publisher's note: The information in this book is not intended as a substitute for
professional medical advice and treatment. If you are pregnant or breastfeeding or have
any special dietary requirements or medical conditions, it is recommended that you consult
a medical professional before following any of the information or recipes contained in this
book. Duncan Baird Publishers, or any other persons who have been involved in working on
this publication, cannot accept responsibility for any errors or omissions, inadvertent or not,
that may be found in the recipes or text, nor for any problems that may arise as a result of
preparing one of these recipes or following the advice contained in this work.

Notes on the recipes
Unless otherwise stated:
• All recipes serve 4
• Use medium eggs, fruit and vegetables
• Use fresh ingredients, including herbs and chillies
• Do not mix metric and imperial measurements
• 1 tsp = 5ml
• 1 tbsp = 15ml
• 1 cup = 250ml

contents

Key to symbols

ANTI-BACTERIAL

ANTIVIRAL

ANTIOXIDANT

ANTI-INFLAMMATORY

ANTI-AGING

ANTI-CANCER

DETOXIFYING

BLOOD-SUGAR BALANCING

ENERGY-BOOSTING

GOOD FOR THE BRAIN

GOOD FOR HAIR, TEETH AND NAILS

GOOD FOR THE SKIN

GOOD FOR THE EYES

GOOD FOR THE HEART

GOOD FOR THE IMMUNE SYSTEM

GOOD FOR THE MUSCULO-SKELETAL SYSTEM

GOOD FOR THE DIGESTIVE SYSTEM

GOOD FOR THE HORMONAL SYSTEM

Introduction

Our ancestors knew well the healing power of natural foods and turned to them to combat all manner of maladies. It's only now, centuries later, that research has begun to confirm that the therapeutic benefits of these foods can be scientifically proven. In fact, some wonderfoods have been found to work even better than drugs – and without the adverse side effects.

Most experts now agree that eating a diet rich in natural, health-giving foods can help us to ward off common complaints such as colds, coughs and infections as well as to protect ourselves against chronic degenerative diseases, including cancer, heart disease and arthritis. So, next time you're feeling below par, instead of turning to the medicine cabinet turn to your own fridge or kitchen cupboard where, with the help of this great book, you're likely to find a remedy.

It really is possible to eat your way to good health and improve the way you feel and look. *Natural Wonderfoods* includes 100 delicious and nutritious foods that you can easily introduce into your diet for maximum impact on your health. The food entries offer practical and reliable information, as well as recipes for tasty dishes, beauty treatments and home remedies (the latter two marked ✳ and ✦ for easy reference), a nutrient list and at-a-glance symbols highlighting each food's health-enhancing properties.

Most fruit and vegetables, especially, have wide-ranging benefits. Many health conditions stem from nutrient deficiencies, so they can be alleviated – and often cured – by eating better. Base your diet on a wide range of vegetables and fruits, backed by wholegrain cereals, organic meat and dairy products, with as little processed food as possible.

Let's take a closer look at the food groups and their nutrients.

FRUITS

Generally fruits contain more vitamins than vegetables, whereas vegetables rate higher in the mineral stakes. Most fruits are exceptionally cleansing and alkalizing, helping to eliminate toxins from the body and to regulate the digestive system by stimulating movement of the digestive tract and improving the body's ability to absorb nutrients. Fruits are also a fantastic source of enzymes, natural sugars and cell-protective phytochemicals.

As the body digests fruits relatively quickly (within 30 minutes), they are best eaten on their own, separately from other foods that take longer to digest. This prevents them from fermenting in the digestive tract. Between meals is probably a good time to fit them in, unless you opt for an all-fruit breakfast.

Both fresh and dried fruits are nutrient-rich, with dried fruits also being an excellent source of minerals. While freshly pressed fruit juices are good for you, it's advisable to dilute them with water to reduce their fruit-sugar content. This will help to curb blood-sugar fluctuations and lower the calorie count, which can add up when fruits are juiced, as well as reduce the risk of dental caries.

VEGETABLES

If there's one food group we can never eat too much of, it has to be vegetables. Abundant in vitamins, minerals, fibre and water, vegetables help to cleanse and alkalize the body, neutralizing acidity and reducing the toxic load. They are also low in fat and calories (with the exception of starchy vegetables, such as potatoes, winter squash and yams) and are one of the best sources of phytochemicals – potent plant compounds that help to protect the body against disease.

Scientific research suggests that phytochemicals slow down the aging process and reduce the risk of diseases, including cancer, heart disease, high blood pressure, osteoporosis and arthritis. Most of them function as antioxidants, helping to counteract the hazardous effects of free radicals – unstable molecules that damage body cells. In fact, free radical damage is thought to be one of the main causes of ageing. Phytochemicals exert various other properties, such as stimulating the immune system, regulating hormones and providing anti-bacterial and antiviral activity. The great news is that all vegetables are full of these natural plant components, of which hundreds have now been identified.

Try to make vegetables a central feature of main meals and find new ways of incorporating them into your diet, so that you eat generous amounts every day. When preparing salads, instead of sticking to basic ingredients such as lettuce, cucumber and tomatoes, use them only as a base, and add a variety of other colourful ingredients such as celery, red pepper, radicchio, beetroot, fennel, watercress and carrots. Cooked vegetables are good too, especially in the winter. To preserve fragile nutrients such as vitamin C, steam, stir-fry or bake them rather than boil them, or add them to soups and stews. Juicing is another great way of reaping the goodness from vegetables in a more concentrated form.

MEAT AND DAIRY

Protein is vital for strong immunity and building strong bones and muscles, as well as essential for repairing the body's tissues, and meat and dairy products abound in it.

This vital component is required to manufacture all cells, including the immune system's antibodies and enzymes. It is made up of amino acids, which play a key role in immune health – for example, the amino acid glutathione is an important antioxidant and detoxifier. Many people are deficient in protein, so we have included protein-rich foods, such as chicken, lamb, eggs and bio-yogurt.

FISH

As well as being a great source of protein, fish, such as sardines, salmon and fresh tuna, are a superb source of the essential fatty acids (EFAs) that play such a vital role in helping us to feel and to look fantastic. Not only do EFAs play a central role in keeping the brain active, the mind agile and the nervous system healthy, but they are also fundamental to the preservation of the elasticity of the skin and to keeping the hair glossy and healthy, and to improving our fitness.

Seafood, such as prawns and oysters, are also loaded with useful minerals, such as iodine, which regulates the thyroid gland, and zinc and selenium, powerful antioxidants that boost immunity and help to fight off infections.

NUTS, SEEDS AND OILS

All these foods provide protein, minerals and vitamin E, which are very important for the skin, reproductive organs and circulatory system. They are also packed with the healthy fats associated with lowering high cholesterol, balancing hormones and reducing inflammation.

The high fat content of nuts and seeds means they are calorie-laden, so eat them in moderation. They are ideal sprinkled on salads, cereals and desserts or as snacks. Also, nut and seed butters make tasty spreads on toast or crackers.

GRAINS, PULSES AND BEANS

Grains are the primary source of energy for many people throughout the world. Unrefined grains are rich in slow-releasing carbohydrates that help sustain and fuel the body. They are also rich in fibre to aid digestion. There are two main types of fibre – soluble and insoluble. Soluble fibre helps to stabilize blood-sugar levels and to lower high cholesterol, while insoluble fibre regulates bowel movements. Grains contain both types.

Some grains, such as quinoa, provide the body with complete protein; other grains need to be combined with beans, pulses or seeds to make their protein more usable by the body. This can easily be achieved and we often do it when preparing meals in traditional combinations – for example, in baked beans on toast, rice and dhal, and so on.

Like fruit and vegetables, grains supply many healing vitamins, minerals and phytochemicals. Most grains supply B-vitamins, which are needed for normal metabolism and a healthy nervous system, along with calcium and magnesium and various trace elements. If you are allergic or intolerant to gluten (a sticky protein found in wheat, rye and oats), there are plenty of grains that are gluten-free, such as rice, millet, buckwheat and quinoa.

Collectively known as legumes, pulses (the edible seeds of certain legumes) and dried beans are an excellent source of protein (especially when combined with grains), as well as soluble and insoluble fibre and complex carbohydrates. This makes them ideal energy foods for balanced blood sugar. They also contain a broad spectrum of minerals and a brain nutrient called lecithin. If legumes cause you to bloat, their gassy effects can be avoided by adding a few bay leaves or a strip of kombu seaweed during the cooking process.

HERBS, SPICES AND OTHERS

Besides adding taste and aroma, herbs and spices boost the nutrient content in all kinds of meals. Some, such as garlic and ginger, are particularly versatile in their culinary uses, while giving fantastic healing and health-enhancing benefits.

To preserve the nutrients of both fresh and dried herbs, add them to dishes toward the end of the cooking time. They also make fabulous substitutes for salt and some aid digestion. However, it's best to add spices earlier to allow their flavour to develop fully. Herbs and spices can be made into medicinal teas to help to relieve various health problems.

There are some foods that do not fit into any of the categories mentioned so far, but without which no book on wonderfoods would be complete. These include condiments, such as cider vinegar, which has long been valued as a curative; the natural sweetener, honey, which also has amazing healing properties; and tofu, which is a low-fat food jam-packed with nutrients, often used in Oriental cuisines.

STORING FOOD

Fresh fruit and vegetables lose much of their vitamin content in storage. So shop where you know food is fresh, keep it in a fridge or a cool place and eat as soon as possible. Fresh meat should be placed on a plate on the bottom shelf of the fridge, where it can't drip onto anything. Fresh herbs can be kept in a clean screwtop jar with a pinch of salt, covered with olive oil, or for a few days in the fridge, wrapped in damp paper.

SUPPLEMENTS

It's always better to get your nutrients from a balanced diet than by taking supplements. No one knows exactly how it works – only that the whole fruit or vegetable seems to provide a full range of nutrients in the right balance. Beta-carotene, for example, is so good for the lungs that smokers who get plenty of it in their diet reduce their risk of lung cancer. Yet taking beta-carotene supplements seems to increase their cancer risk. It's almost impossible to overdose on nutrients from fruit and vegetables, but it's easy to unbalance your levels of vitamins, and especially minerals, if you take them in the large quantities supplied by supplements. The only exception is vitamin B12. Vegans who can't get enough of this from their diet should take this as part of a vitamin B-complex supplement.

EAT ORGANIC

Organic foods are produced in much the same way food was grown for thousands of years, until the twentieth century. Organic farmers don't use synthetic chemicals or sewage sludge. Their animals are given medicines only when they're unwell – not to make them put on weight faster or as a way of counteracting the unhealthy conditions of factory farms. It's worth paying a little extra to eat organic, although the price difference is narrowing all the time. Not all scientific studies have found that organic foods are more nutritious, but many have – and none has found them less healthy!

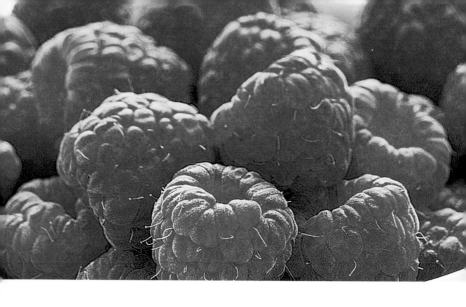

SWEET, SOUR, TANGY OR
JUICY, FRUIT IS NOT ONLY
DELICIOUS, IT'S PACKED
WITH VITAL NUTRIENTS
THAT HELP YOUR BODY
TO FUNCTION AT ITS BEST

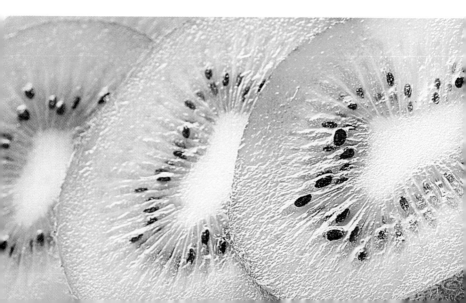

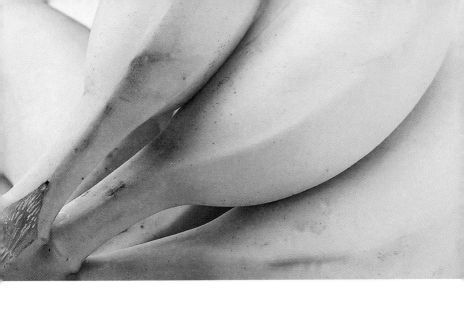

01 | **wonder**
FRUITS

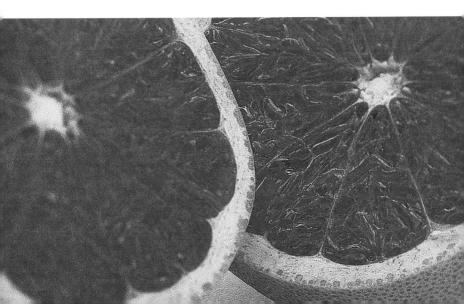

Lemon

VITAMINS B3, B5, B6, C, E, BETA-CAROTENE, BIOTIN, FOLIC ACID; CALCIUM,
COPPER, IODINE, IRON, MAGNESIUM, MANGANESE, PHOSPHORUS, POTASSIUM,
SELENIUM, ZINC; LIMONENE; FLAVONOIDS; FIBRE; CARBOHYDRATE

**Arguably the most versatile of all fruits, the lemon
contains a wealth of health-enhancing properties.
Used originally by the Romans to sweeten the breath,
the lemon is packed full of nutrients and is used today
to treat a number of ailments.**

Like other citrus fruits, lemons are powerhouses of antioxidant vitamin
C, which helps to boost the immune system, assist the healing of wounds
and strengthen the walls of blood capillaries. The high level of vitamin C
in lemons also means that they are vital for healthy skin and gums. They
are a good source of flavonoids, such as quercetin, which boost the
effects of vitamin C, and are particularly important for the health of
blood vessels and to prevent varicose veins.

Lemons contain limonene, a chemical that has been shown to slow
the rate of cancer growth. Limonene also has antiseptic qualities to help
to kill germs – one of the reasons that lemons are traditionally used as
a gargle for sore throats and to treat infections of the respiratory tract.
Lemons also have powerful antifungal properties. They are a popular
ingredient in beauty products, such as skin cleansers and hair conditioners, because, when used in treatments, lemon juice inhibits bacterial
growth and is astringent, strengthening and toning. The fruit's dissolving and extracting qualities can also help in the topical treatment of skin
infections, such as boils and abscesses.

As lemons are a liver stimulant, they can be used for detoxification
purposes. Despite the sourness of lemon juice, it is a popular drink when
diluted in water, with a cleansing taste few other fruits can match. During a brief detox fast, it quells the appetite and freshens breath. Being
one of the most concentrated food sources of vitamin C also makes it
the ideal addition to a glass of water to help soothe a post-exercise dry
throat. Or try diluting freshly squeezed lemon juice with warm water
and drinking it on an empty stomach first thing in the morning to give

your metabolism a kick-start. (However, take care not to drink the juice too often as it can have a detrimental effect on tooth enamel.)

Lemons stimulate the gall bladder, which in turn aids liver and digestive function. Citric acid, which encourages healthy digestion, makes up 7 to 8 per cent of a lemon, the highest concentration found in any fruit. Used in a marinade or salad dressing, lemon juice tenderizes and breaks down some of the tough components of meat. Its calming effect on the stomach relieves bloating and heartburn. Lemons also have a slightly antibacterial effect, reducing the risk of discomfort in the intestines.

The health-giving properties of lemons can be utilized in many ways. The fruits make a great flavouring agent in drinks and foods, from baked goods to sauces. Their juice can be sprinkled onto peeled fruit, such as apples and bananas, to stop them from turning brown, and their zest and pith can be added to casseroles, stews and soups to give extra nutrients.

ZESTY LEMON DRESSING *serves 2*

60ml/2fl oz lemon juice
185ml /6fl oz tomato juice
1 clove garlic , crushed
1 tsp wholegrain mustard
grated zest of 1 lemon

Add all the ingredients, apart from the lemon zest, to a jar with a screw top and shake well. Pour into a bowl and add the zest, blending in with a fork. Drizzle immediately over a salad.

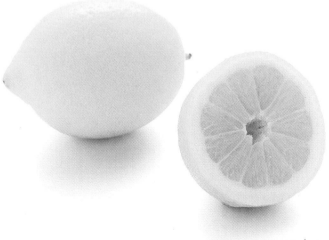

✦LEMON POULTICE *for boils & abscesses*

1 lemon, sliced
gauze bandage

Use the bandage to tie a slice of
lemon against the boil or abscess.
A hot-water bottle can be used to
apply heat, if desired. Leave for about
10 minutes, then discard. Repeat
2 or 3 times a day until the boil
opens and drains.

✦LEMON TONER *to treat thread veins*

4 tsp vegetable glycerin
juice of 1 lemon
1 drop neroli essential oil
1 drop rose essential oil

Mix the vegetable glycerin with the
lemon juice and add the essential
oils. Apply twice daily to thread
veins. Keeps in a sealed jar for up
to 3 months.

TANGY FISH

4 skinless tuna or other
   fish fillets
juice and grated zest of 1 lemon
juice and grated zest of 1 lime
2 tbsp olive oil
2 tsp finely chopped chives
1 tsp ground black pepper

Preheat the grill and place the fish on
a foil-lined grill pan. Mix the zests
with the oil and coat each fish fillet.
Grill for around 8–10 minutes, until
cooked through, turning once. Mix
together the juices, chives and
pepper. Pour the mixture over
the fish and serve immediately.

LEMONADE

750ml/26fl oz/3 cups carbonated water
600ml/21fl oz/2⅓ cups white grape juice
juice of 3 lemons
1 tbsp agave syrup

Put all the ingredients in a glass
pitcher and stir. Serve chilled with
plenty of ice.

LEMONY STUFFING BALLS *makes 10 balls*

1 small onion, quartered

1 egg, beaten

1 tbsp chopped rosemary

125g/4½oz/1½ cups fresh white breadcrumbs

juice and grated zest of 1 lemon

Whizz the onion, egg and rosemary in a blender until smooth. In a bowl, mix the breadcrumbs with the lemon juice and zest, then combine the mixtures together. Form into 10 small balls. Place on a baking tray and bake in a preheated oven at 180˚C/350˚F/ gas mark 4 for 25 minutes. Serve as an accompaniment.

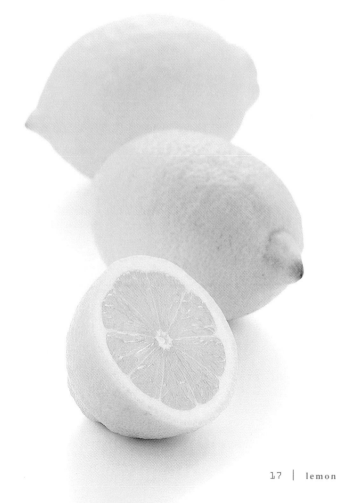

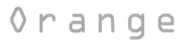

Orange

VITAMINS A, B1, B3, B5, C, E, K, BETA-CAROTENE, FOLIC ACID; BETA-SITOSTEROL; CALCIUM, IODINE, IRON, MAGNESIUM, PHOSPHORUS, POTASSIUM, SELENIUM, ZINC; LIMONENE, HESPERIDIN; FIBRE

Native to Asia, oranges are high in vitamin C and fibre, and rich in natural sugars for quick energy. Highly popular, they contain many disease-fighting compounds.

Oranges are one of the top sources of vitamin C, which is crucial for strong immunity, helping to fight viruses and produce disease-fighting cells to battle bacteria. A medium-sized orange provides more than the average daily requirement of vitamin C, which can also help to reduce post-exercise muscle soreness. Particularly effective against colds, flu and other respiratory ailments, including asthma, oranges have also been found to reduce the risk of stomach ulcers and kidney stones.

They contain beta-sitosterol, a plant sterol that helps to prevent tumour formation. In addition, oranges are rich in vitamin B5, which helps to stimulate the body's immune response, and are loaded with fibre, needed for a healthy heart and digestive system. High in the antioxidant hesperidin, oranges are said to protect the heart further by raising healthy HDL cholesterol and lowering "bad" LDL cholesterol, and to stop harmful free radicals from clogging up the arteries – a key risk factor for heart disease.

The wealth of vitamins and minerals found in oranges help to maintain healthy, youthful skin, and prevent eye problems. The fruits also contain limonene, a compound that has anti-carcinogenic properties. Their natural sugars help diabetics to maintain their blood-glucose levels. Oranges are even reputed to reduce cellulite.

TANGY PANCAKES

1 egg
150ml/5fl oz/scant ⅔ cup
  skimmed milk
70g/2½oz/scant ⅔ cup plain flour
grated zest of 1 orange
2 oranges
1 tbsp sugar
15g/½oz unsalted butter
4 tbsp plain bio-yogurt to serve

Beat together the egg and milk, then fold in the flour and zest of one orange. Peel both the oranges, and divide them into segments. Put the orange segments in a saucepan. Add the sugar, and cook over a low heat for 2 minutes. Melt a little butter in a frying pan, then add a quarter of the batter mixture for each pancake, cooking until golden brown, turning once. Serve with the oranges and the yogurt.

ORANGE YOGURT SUNDAE

4 tbsp plain bio-yogurt
grated zest of ½ orange
2 oranges, peeled and sliced into wheels
1 banana, sliced
1 tbsp berries of your choice
¼ tsp cinnamon

Mix together the yogurt and the zest and chill for an hour. In a separate bowl, mix together the fruit and cinnamon and chill. Divide the fruit salad into bowls and spoon the yogurt over. Serve immediately.

CHOCOLATE ORANGES

100g/3½oz plain chocolate, grated
1 tbsp golden syrup
grated zest of 1 orange
4 tbsp single cream
4 oranges, peeled

Put the grated chocolate and syrup in a heatproof bowl and melt gently over a pan of simmering water. Once they have melted, turn off the heat and stir in the zest and cream. Divide the oranges into segments and arrange them on plates. Drizzle over the sauce and serve.

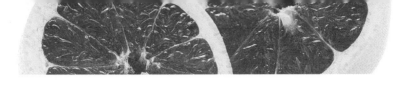

Grapefruit

Vitamin B3, B5, C, E, beta-carotene, biotin, folic acid, lycopene;
calcium, iodine, iron, magnesium, phosphorus, potassium; flavonoids;
liminoids; fibre; carbohydrate

The perfect breakfast food, grapefruit is loaded with antioxidants and is a powerful detoxifier.

The grapefruit is thought to have originated in the Caribbean island of Jamaica, before reaching the rest of the world in the eighteenth century. There are several different varieties, including yellow, pink and ruby-red types. The pink and red varieties are coloured by lycopene, a carotenoid with heart-protective and anti-cancer properties. These are also sweeter in taste and are therefore the best option for anyone who dislikes the more tangy flavour of the white variety. The fruit is delicious cut in half so that the flesh can be scooped out, and simply eaten on its own, or drizzled with a little honey. It also works well juiced, either alone or in combination with other fruit, such as apple or raspberries, although juicing removes the benefits offered by its fibre content.

The high vitamin-C content of grapefruit enhances immunity, helping to reduce and relieve colds, heal cuts and reduce bruising, and it also has anti-aging properties. The pink variety, in particular, is a good source of potassium and bioflavonoids, both of which are important for the heart and circulation, as well as the skin and immunity. Bioflavonoids also strengthen blood capillaries. The fruit's seeds contain an anti-parasite, anti-fungal compound which, although not edible whole, can be taken in supplement form (grapefruit seed extract). Grapefruit is also rich in alpha-hydroxy-acids (AHAs), which make it an effective toner when used topically.

Every part of a grapefruit is a powerful detoxifier. Its flesh and zest are thought to contain compounds that help to inhibit cancer development. The pulp is high in pectin, a soluble fibre that binds with excess cholesterol to remove it from the body, and helps to eliminate toxins.

Consuming a grapefruit first thing in the morning can kick-start the digestive system and relieve constipation, while starting a meal with grapefruit is an old diet trick that does seem to work. In a study in 2006, scientists found that this simple action helped some very overweight volunteers to lose weight. Their blood-sugar levels were healthier than usual afterwards, too. Other evidence suggests that eating grapefruit can steady insulin levels. So these nutrient-rich fruits could help to prevent the vicious cycle in which gaining weight leads to diabetes, and diabetes makes people put on even more weight.

STUFFED GRAPEFRUIT

2 grapefruit, halved, flesh removed and chopped
1 avocado, pitted, peeled and cubed
2.5cm/1in piece root ginger, chopped
1 pear, peeled, cored and cubed
1 green pepper, deseeded and chopped
2 black olives, pitted and halved
2 tbsp lemon balm, finely chopped

Mix the grapefruit flesh with the avocado, ginger, pear and green pepper, and divide the filling among the 4 halves. Garnish with the olives and lemon balm, and serve.

GRAPEFRUIT AND CHICKEN SALAD

grated zest of 2 grapefruit
4 tbsp honey vinaigrette (see p.271)
350g/12oz/2 cups cooked chicken, shredded
2 grapefruit, unpeeled and cut into wheels
4 sweet peppers, deseeded and cut into rings

Add the grapefruit zest to the vinaigrette. Pour it over the chicken pieces. Put the grapefruit wheels and the pepper rings into a dish and pile the chicken on top.

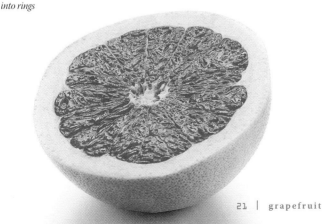

*GRAPEFRUIT BEAUTY MASK *to tone the skin*

1 small grapefruit, peeled and broken
  into segments
1 small pot natural yogurt

Remove the pith and pips from the grapefruit segments and put them with the yogurt in a blender. Whizz to make a paste. Put the mixture in a bowl and leave in the fridge for 1 hour. Apply to the face and leave for about 10 minutes. Gently remove with cool water.

CITRUS FRUIT SALAD

3 large handfuls mixed salad leaves
2 tbsp chopped parsley
1 tbsp chopped coriander
1 tbsp sunflower seeds
½ pink grapefruit
1 tbsp olive oil
1 tbsp lemon juice
1 tbsp orange juice

Put the salad leaves, parsley, coriander and sunflower seeds in a large bowl. Cut the grapefruit into segments and add them to the bowl. Drizzle the olive oil and citrus juices over the salad, then toss gently and serve immediately.

HONEY-MARINATED GRAPEFRUIT

4 ruby grapefruit
2 tbsp honey
1 tbsp chopped fresh mint

Squeeze the juice of 1 grapefruit and grate 1 teaspoon of the zest; set aside. Warm the honey in a pan. Add the juice and zest. Mix well. Peel the 3 remaining grapefruit and separate into segments. Arrange on a plate and cover with the marinade. Leave to stand for 15 minutes. Sprinkle with the mint.

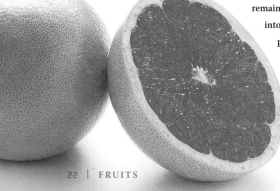

Banana

VITAMINS B2, B3, B5, B6, C, K, BETA-CAROTENE, BIOTIN, FOLIC ACID; CALCIUM, COPPER, IODINE, IRON, MAGNESIUM, MANGANESE, PHOSPHORUS, POTASSIUM, SELENIUM, ZINC; FIBRE; CARBOHYDRATE; TRYPTOPHAN

The ultimate fast food, bananas provide a potent mix of vitamins, minerals and carbohydrates.

A banana is often a favourite fruit of babies and children and in adult life can trigger feelings of being safe and nurtured. Rich in healthy carbohydrates, bananas are ideal when you crave comfort foods, as they feel enjoyably self-indulgent and they're stuffed with nutrients that soothe and lift your mood. They contain tryptophan, which the body converts to serotonin to ease depression and promote peaceful sleep.

Bananas contain high levels of B-vitamins, which the body needs to produce energy. These include vitamin B5, which aids the formation of the immune system's killer cells, and B6, which improves the body's ability to clear away waste matter and reduces fatigue and premenstrual symptoms. Bananas are also a good source of immunity-enhancing vitamin C, and contain manganese, which works with this vitamin to produce the virus-fighting substance interferon. In addition, they are high in potassium, which regulates body fluids and nerve function.

As well as maintaining healthy nerve and muscle function, bananas lower blood pressure and protect against heart disease by maintaining fluid balance and preventing plaque from sticking to artery walls. They are also rich in fibre, and are therefore highly beneficial to the digestive tract, soothing and helping to restore normal function after constipation or diarrhoea. Bananas contain FOS (fructo-oligo-saccharides), which help to feed "good" bacteria in the gut and to aid digestion, and they act as antacids, useful for heartburn or ulcers.

Ripe bananas contain the ideal carbohydrate combination to replace muscle glycogen before or during exercise, making them a valuable food for athletes. Glucose, the most easily digested sugar, is immediately absorbed into the bloodstream for instant energy, while the fructose in bananas is absorbed more slowly, providing a steady supply of fuel over time. Banana skins can soften corns and calluses.

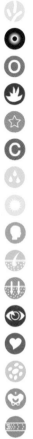

GRILLED BANANAS WITH LIME SYRUP

serves 2

115g/4oz sugar
juice and grated zest of 2 limes
100ml/3½fl oz/scant 1 cup water
4 bananas, sliced into chunks

Put half the sugar in a saucepan with the lime juice and zest, and the water. Bring to the boil, reduce the heat and simmer for 10 minutes until thick. Place the bananas on some foil, sprinkle with the remaining sugar, and grill, turning occasionally, until golden and soft. Drizzle with the lime syrup, and serve.

✦ BANANA SKIN POULTICE *for corns & calluses*

2 small, unripe banana skins
strip of cloth

Using the cloth, bandage a piece of unripe banana skin, gummy-side down, onto the corn or callus. Leave overnight and discard in the morning. Repeat the following night. After 2 days soak the feet in hot water, then scrape away the softened corn with a pumice stone. Repeat as necessary.

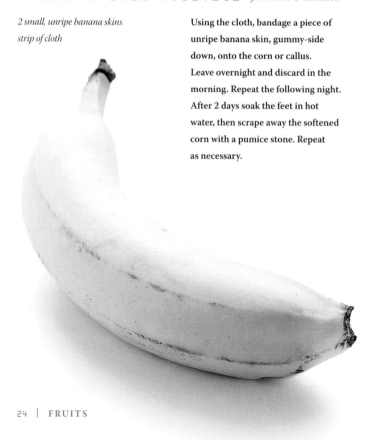

*BANANA CONDITIONER *to moisturize dry hair*

1 ripe banana
2 tsp grapeseed oil

Mash the banana using a fork, then mix with the oil to make a paste. Massage into the hair and scalp, then cover the hair with cling film and leave for 30 minutes. Wash out using a mild shampoo.

SPICED BANANAS

4 bananas, peeled
4 tsp lemon juice
2 tsp ground cinnamon
2 tbsp flaked almonds

Slice the bananas in half lengthways and place on an oiled baking sheet. Sprinkle with the lemon juice and cinnamon and place under a hot grill until the bananas start to brown. Scatter the almonds over, and serve.

BREAKFAST SMOOTHIE *serves 2*

2 ripe bananas
20 raspberries
20 blueberries
500g/1lb 2oz/2 cups plain bio-yogurt
½ tsp ground ginger

Whizz together the bananas, berries and yogurt in a blender until smooth. Pour into two glasses, sprinkle over the ginger and serve immediately.

BANANA MILKSHAKE

2 bananas, chopped
500ml/17fl oz/2 cups soya milk or milk
  of your choice
1 tbsp maple syrup
1 tbsp natural vanilla extract
1 tsp ground nutmeg

Put the bananas, milk, maple syrup and vanilla extract in a blender and whizz until smooth. Serve chilled, sprinkled with the nutmeg.

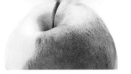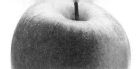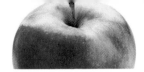

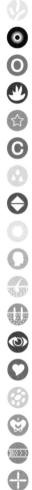

Apple

VITAMINS B3, C, E, K, BETA-CAROTENE, BIOTIN, FOLIC ACID; CALCIUM, CHROMIUM, IRON, MAGNESIUM, MANGANESE, PHOSPHORUS, POTASSIUM, ZINC; MALIC ACID, QUERCETIN; FLAVONOIDS; FIBRE; CARBOHYDRATE

Over the course of centuries, apple has acquired a reputation as a healthful fruit and remedy, so confirming the old adage, "An apple a day keeps the doctor away."

Apples have a huge number of health benefits, and scientists are only just starting to identify their numerous life-enhancing nutrients, but their superstar role is in digestion and detoxification. Eating an apple aids a detox by helping you feel full sooner and for longer, and can alleviate even chronic constipation, a widespread problem often caused by poor nutrition. Constipation prevents the body getting rid of toxins and can lead to more serious conditions, from haemorrhoids to colon cancer.

Apples are rich in soluble and insoluble fibre, both of which help food to progress at a healthy pace through the digestive system. These fibres pick up toxic waste, such as heavy metals, along the way, as well as cholesterol, which is one reason why apples are also good for the arteries. The toxins and cholesterol can then be safely excreted, with the help of the soluble fibre, pectin. It forms a gel-like substance that softens

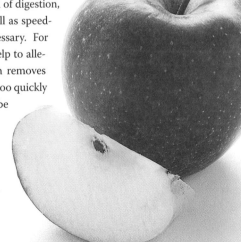

the body's waste and helps it to leave the body naturally. Pectin has a regulating effect on the speed of digestion, slowing it down as well as speeding it up when necessary. For example, it can also help to alleviate diarrhoea, which removes food from the system too quickly for vital nutrients to be absorbed and can lead to dangerous levels of dehydration.

Apples also contain malic acid, which

neutralizes acid by-products and helps the body to use energy efficiently. They slow the rise of blood sugar and help to control diabetes. Studies have found that eating them can even help to improve lung function.

According to studies, apples may reduce the risk of several common cancers, as well as protect the brain from the damage that causes conditions such as Alzheimer's and Parkinson's disease. Antioxidant compounds in the skin of apples, in particular quercetin, epicatechin and procyanidin, are thought to be responsible for this protective action. Quercetin is also an anti-inflammatory, making apples useful in the treatment of arthritis and allergic reactions, and reducing the risk of sun damage to skin. The vitamin C content of apples boosts immunity, while their high water content rehydrates the body.

BAKED APPLES *serves 2*

55g/2oz unsalted butter

4 tsp currants

4 tsp sugar

4 tsp flaked almonds

1 tsp ground cinnamon

1 tsp ground nutmeg

2 cooking apples, peeled and cored

2 tbsp natural fromage frais, to serve

Preheat the oven to 180°C/350°F/gas mark 4. Combine all the ingredients, apart from the apples, in a bowl. Divide the mixture in half and stuff into each apple. Wrap the apples individually in foil, and bake for 20 minutes. Serve topped with fromage frais.

✦ AGE-OLD APPLE AND LICORICE INFUSION
for gastric, kidney & pulmonary conditions

2kg/4½lb apples, unpeeled
  and thinly sliced into rounds

1l/35fl oz/4 cups water

2 small pieces licorice root

Place the apples in a saucepan and cover with the water. Add the licorice root and boil for 15 minutes, then strain and discard the apple and licorice. Drink throughout the day.

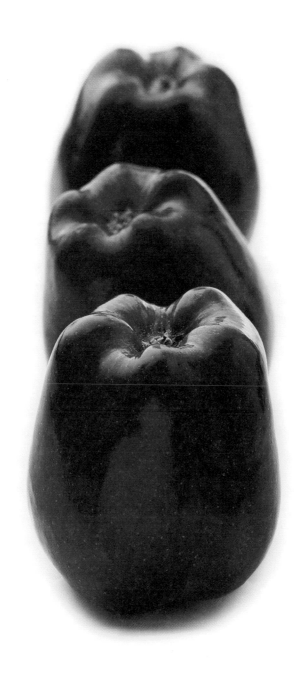

APPLE, PEAR AND MINT JUICE

8 apples, cored
8 pears, cored
12 stems mint

Wash all the fruit, then cut it into chunks, leaving the skin on. Feed through a juicer with the mint. Pour into large glasses and drink immediately.

APPLE CHARLOTTE

1kg/2lb 4oz cooking apples, peeled, cored
  and sliced
2 tbsp honey
½ tsp ground cinnamon
pinch of nutmeg
8 slices of bread, buttered on both sides

Preheat the oven to 190°C/ 375°F/ gas mark 5. Heat the apples with 2 tablespoons of water in a pan, stirring until the mixture forms a thick purée. Stir in the honey, cinnamon and nutmeg. Line the sides and base of a greased cake tin with half the bread, spoon the purée in and top with the other half. Bake for 30 minutes, until golden brown. Serve immediately.

APPLE AND APRICOT CRUMBLE

200ml/7fl oz/¾ cup apple juice
6 apples, peeled, cored and chopped
280g/10oz apricot jam
55g/2oz unhydrogenated margarine
115g/4oz/1 cup rolled oats
3 tbsp oatbran

Put the apple juice in a pan and bring to the boil. Add the apples and simmer, covered, until the liquid is absorbed. Mash, add the jam, and spread in an oven-proof dish. Work the margarine into the oats and oatbran to form a crumble. Spoon it over the fruit and bake at 180°C/ 350°F/gas mark 4 for 30 minutes.

Pear

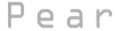

Vitamins B3, C, E, K, beta-carotene, biotin, folic acid; calcium, copper, iodine, iron, magnesium, phosphorus, potassium, zinc; fibre; carbohydrate

Sweet and satisfying, pears are rich in fibre, which can help the body to shed excess weight. Besides making an ideal dessert or snack, pears and pear juice can be used to sweeten cakes and cereals instead of sugar.

Both soluble and insoluble fibre help to fill you up in a healthy way. Pears are among the few fruits that contain a high quantity of insoluble fibre, which works like tiny scrubbing brushes in the colon to promote good digestion. Their sweet taste and refreshing juiciness make them an appealing option to anyone who has given up sugary treats in order to lose weight. Also, when people are trying to lose weight, the change in diet sometimes disturbs the eliminatory system. Pears counteract any tendency towards sluggish digestion if you're eating less than usual.

Pears are often given as a baby's first fruit, as they are the least likely to cause an allergic reaction. This also makes them one of the best fruits for people with multiple food allergies. The insoluble fibre in pears helps to eliminate cholesterol from the body, which is useful for those at risk of heart disease. The antioxidant vitamin C and folic acid content in pears also boost immunity and help to fight off infections.

One pear contains roughly one-tenth of the recommended daily potassium intake for most adults – a mineral lost through perspiration. This means that pears make great snacks for exercisers, as they counteract the low potassium levels that can lead to fatigue and muscle cramps.

GRILLED PEARS

4 pears, halved and cored
2 tbsp currants
4 tbsp apple juice

Grill the pears under a low heat for 5 minutes, turning once. Sprinkle the currants on top and pour over the apple juice. Serve immediately.

PEARS IN CAROB

300ml/10½fl oz/1¼ cups white grape juice
6 pears, peeled, cored and cut in half
   lengthways
280g/10oz silken tofu
3 tbsp brown rice syrup
2 tbsp hazelnut butter
1 tsp carob powder
1 tsp grain coffee substitute
2 tbsp sunflower oil

Put two-thirds of the grape juice in a pan and bring to the boil. Add the pears, reduce the heat and simmer, covered, for 8 minutes until the liquid has evaporated. Divide into four dessert bowls. Put the remaining juice and ingredients in a food processor and whizz until creamy. Serve with the cooked pears.

POACHED PEARS

4 pears, peeled
100g/3½oz clear honey
125ml/4½fl oz/½ cup
   apple juice
1 tsp ground ginger

Place the pears in a pan. Pour over the honey, juice and 250ml/9fl oz/1 cup water. Sprinkle over the ginger and bring to the boil. Reduce the heat and simmer, covered, for 20 minutes. Allow to cool in the syrup.

Fig

VITAMINS B3, B5, B6, C, BETA-CAROTENE, BIOTIN, FOLIC ACID; CALCIUM, COPPER, IODINE, IRON, MAGNESIUM, MANGANESE, PHOSPHORUS, POTASSIUM, ZINC; FIBRE; CARBOHYDRATE

Nature's own laxative, figs are indigenous to Iran, Syria and other parts of Asia, and are generously high in health-enhancing compounds.

Figs contain active ingredients that stimulate the intestinal action necessary for bowel movement, relieving constipation, which is often a problem in later life. They also contain more fibre than any other dried or fresh fruit, aiding satiety by promoting a feeling of fullness in the stomach and helping to balance blood-sugar levels. In addition, their high fibre content provides a further laxative effect.

Two of the minerals found in figs help to protect the skeletal system: calcium, vital for bone growth in children and bone density in adults, and potassium, which also helps to control the blood pressure and water-balance in the body.

Calcium is particularly important for female athletes who train at high intensity. This is because they may experience low oestrogen levels and amenorrhoea, which can increase bone loss and the need for calcium. Most of us eat too much sodium (mainly from salt) and not enough potassium, which balances some of sodium's effects. While excess sodium causes the body to excrete calcium, potassium helps to reduce this loss. It also counteracts sodium's harmful effects on blood pressure and lowers the risk of developing heart conditions. Figs are also rich in iron, needed to stave off anaemia, making them an excellent food for pregnant women and convalescents.

Dried figs offer a concentrated burst of simple carbohydrate for instant energy – Spartan athletes in ancient Greece were said to eat figs to boost their performance – while fresh figs provide a unique, sweet taste and crunchy texture, and a higher dose of the vital antioxidant vitamin C. Figs also provide useful amounts of vitamin B6, without which we can suffer from a poor memory and increased stress levels. Used topically, they are good at drawing out poisons.

✦ FIG SYRUP *for constipation*

55g/2oz/⅓ cup dried figs
55g/2oz/⅓ cup prunes
455ml/16fl oz/scant 2 cups water
1 tbsp treacle

Put the figs, prunes and water in a saucepan. Soak for 8 hours, then bring to the boil, reduce heat and simmer until the fruit is soft and the excess liquid has reduced. Stir in the treacle, then cool and whizz in a food processor. Transfer to a jam jar and store in the refrigerator. Take 1 dessertspoon of the syrup as needed.

FIGS STUFFED WITH ORANGE-ANISE CREAM

16 dried figs
115g/4 oz cream cheese,
  at room temperature
1 tbsp fresh orange juice
2 tsp grated orange zest
1½ tsp clear honey
½ tsp aniseed, crushed

Trim and discard the stems from the figs. Cut an "X" down through the stem ends and gently push each fig open. In a bowl combine the cream cheese, orange juice, orange zest, honey and aniseed. Beat until creamy. Spoon a dollop of mixture into each fig. Keeps in the fridge for 2 hours.

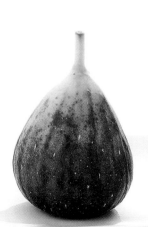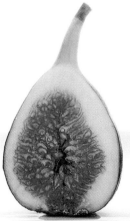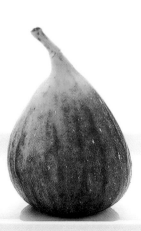

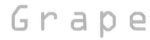

Grape

Vitamins B1, B3, B6, C, K, beta-carotene, biotin, folic acid; calcium, copper, iodine, iron, magnesium, manganese, phosphorus, potassium, selenium, zinc; anthocyanins, ellagic acid, flavonoids, quercetin; fibre; carbohydrate

These sweet and juicy vine fruits are nature's cleansers and make excellent detoxifiers. A great source of instant energy, succulent grapes provide all-round protection.

Grapes contain an enormous number of compounds that are uniquely nourishing, thus giving them a reputation as a food for convalescents. This aromatic fruit can prevent and help to treat any number of age-related conditions, from anaemia and fatigue to arthritis, varicose veins and rheumatism.

Since the earliest times, grapes have been dried to make raisins. Dynamos of concentrated nutrients, raisins are full of fibre and are an exceptionally high-energy food. They are also rich in the minerals iron, potassium, selenium and zinc. Selenium, in particular, is a very important anti-aging nutrient, offering protection from heart disease and boosting the immune system. In addition, selenium is good for the skin and is thought to help keep fine lines and wrinkles at bay.

In folk medicine, grapes were used to purify the blood, clean the digestive system and counter liver and kidney disorders. Their high vitamin C content means that they are helpful for mopping up harmful free radicals, and being high in both water and fibre, grapes are a great aid for detoxifying the skin, gut, kidneys and the liver.

Full of powerful antioxidants, including astringent tannins, flavonids and anthocyanins, grapes help to prevent "bad" LDL cholesterol from oxidizing and blood from clotting, and strengthen capillaries, therefore protecting the heart and the circulatory system. Black grapes also contain quercetin, which helps to minimize inflammation, aiding the cardiovascular system further, as well as promoting healthy digestion.

Grapes can help to stabilize immune response by moderating allergic reactions. They also contain cancer-preventing ellagic acid as well as resveratrol, which is found specifically in red grapes. This compound, together with pterostilbene and saponins, aids heart health by reducing the risk of blood clots and relaxing blood vessels.

When fitting in food before exercise is a problem, grapes provide a refreshing solution. Grapes make an ideal pre-workout snack, as they are light, rich in quick-energy carbohydrate and easily digestible, and they replenish some of the fluid and minerals you'll lose as you sweat. It helps if you can keep them in your pocket and nibble them as you go along.

GRAPE CLEANSER *serves 1–2*

20 seedless grapes
6 celery stalks
1 handful watercress

Press the ingredients through a juicer, alternating the grapes, celery and watercress. Mix well and drink immediately.

GRAPE JUICE

2.7kg/6lb black grapes
piece of muslin

Place the grapes in a large stockpot. Mash them so that the juice flows. Cover them with water and bring to the boil, then reduce the heat to simmer for 10 minutes. Mash them again, breaking up as many grapes as possible. Then, secure the muslin over another pot and pour the juice through it. Allow the juice to stand overnight. Remove the muslin and drink.

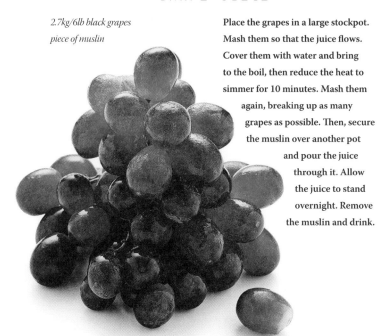

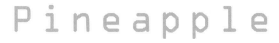

Pineapple

Vitamins B1, B2, B3, B5, B6, C, E, K, beta-carotene, biotin, folic acid;
copper, iron, magnesium, manganese, phosphorus, potassium, zinc;
bromelain, fibre

**Not only a delicious exotic fruit, pineapple also has
a special health asset in the form of bromelain, an enzyme
that helps in the digestion of protein and can reduce
inflammation and swelling throughout the body.**

In ancient Indian medicine, pineapples were thought to act as a uterine tonic, but today they are best known for their anti-inflammatory action. The enzyme bromelain found in fresh pineapple is a protein-digesting enzyme that aids the digestive system and inhibits the action of a number of inflammatory agents, thereby easing inflammatory conditions such as sinusitis, rheumatoid arthritis and gout, speeding recovery from injuries and surgery, helping to alleviate fluid retention and preventing blood clots and conditions such as arteriosclerosis. Bromelain can also help the gut to operate efficiently and effectively, and is therefore a useful remedy for digestive problems.

Pineapple is an excellent source of manganese – an essential cofactor in a number of enzymes important for antioxidant defences and energy production and needed for skin, bone and cartilage formation. In addition, pineapple is rich in antioxidant vitamin C, which supports the immune system and defends against damaging free radicals, which can cause premature aging. Vitamin C, along with manganese also helps to make bone-protecting collagen. Used topically, pineapple can help to soften and remove dead skin through the action of its enzyme bromelain.

PINEAPPLE AND CUCUMBER SALAD

300g/10½oz large cucumber,
   peeled and thinly sliced
a pinch of salt
300g/10½oz pineapple, peeled, cored
   and chopped
2 tbsp mayonnaise mixed with
   lemon juice
mint leaves, to serve

Put the cucumber in a colander, sprinkle with salt and leave for 20 minutes. Rinse off the salt and squeeze out the water. Mix the cucumber and pineapple in a bowl. Chill for 2 hours, then add the mayonnaise and toss well. Garnish with mint leaves to serve.

PINEAPPLE AND HONEY MARINADE
for salmon or chicken

200g/7oz pineapple, peeled, cored
   and finely chopped
2 garlic cloves, crushed
1–2 tbsp clear honey
1 tsp ground allspice
1 tsp ground nutmeg
1 tsp ground cinnamon
1 tsp ground cloves
a pinch of salt

Mix together all the ingredients and leave to stand for 15 minutes. Pour over the salmon or chicken and leave to marinate for 2 hours before cooking.

PINEAPPLE AND MANGO SALSA

1 large mango
½ pineapple
¼ red onion, chopped
1cm/½in piece root ginger, peeled and
   grated
1 garlic clove, crushed
½ red chilli, deseeded and finely sliced
1 handful coriander, roughly chopped
juice of 2 limes
1 tsp sesame oil

Peel and chop the flesh of the fruits, then put it in a bowl with the onion, ginger, garlic, chilli and coriander. Toss well. Drizzle the lime juice and sesame oil on to the mixture. Serve with fish or chicken, or as a dip.

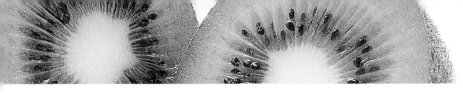

Kiwi fruit

VITAMINS B3, B5, B6, C, E, BETA-CAROTENE, BIOTIN, FOLIC ACID; LUTEIN; CALCIUM, COPPER, IODINE, IRON, MAGNESIUM, MANGANESE, PHOSPHORUS, POTASSIUM, SELENIUM, ZINC; FIBRE; CARBOHYDRATE

Named after an indigenous New Zealand bird, kiwi fruit is a top immunity booster containing more vitamin C than oranges.

The immunity-enhancing abilities of the kiwi fruit lie mainly in its super-dose of vitamin C. Just one fruit contains around 120 per cent of an adult's daily recommended intake, and unlike many other fruits, the nutrients remain intact long after harvesting, with 90 per cent of its vitamin C content still present after 6 months' storage. And although vitamin C is well known for warding off colds, its effects go much further than that. It protects the body from all kinds of infections and inflammation, and is particularly effective against respiratory diseases. Scientists have found that it helps to reduce coughing, wheezing and rhinitis. In addition, people who eat kiwi fruit are less likely than others to suffer from asthma attacks. However, the fruit shouldn't be given to very small children as it can sometimes cause allergies.

Kiwi fruit are loaded with lutein, a carotene, which, together with vitamins C and E, helps to reduce blood clotting as well as blood fats. Their high levels of vitamins C and E are particularly good for preserving youthful skin and protecting vision, and being potassium-rich, kiwis can prevent many age-related conditions from high blood pressure to insomnia and exhaustion.

A good source of fibre, kiwi fruit have mild laxative qualities, which help to promote an efficient digestive system. In helping to eliminate toxins from the body, kiwis also help to lower cholesterol levels, which enhances heart health. Phytonutrients in kiwis have been found to have an anti-thrombotic effect, which is good news for people who are at high risk of heart disease and strokes. According to research, blood clotting was significantly reduced in those consuming two to three kiwi fruit a day. With further studies, this fruit could possibly become a natural alternative to aspirin as a blood-thinning agent.

KIWI AND AVOCADO SALAD

3 kiwi fruit, peeled and sliced
2 avocados, pitted, peeled and sliced
1 apple, cored and sliced
2 tsp lemon juice
3 tbsp olive oil
1 tbsp wine vinegar
100g/3½oz lettuce, shredded

Place 2 of the kiwi fruit, the avocados, apple and lemon juice in a bowl and mix together. Crush the remaining kiwi fruit, then blend with the olive oil and vinegar. Pour the mixture over the fruit and toss again. Serve on a bed of lettuce.

KIWI FRUIT ICE

4 kiwi fruit, peeled and chopped
500ml/17fl oz/2 cups unsweetened
   apple juice
1 tbsp lemon juice
½ tsp grated orange rind

Combine the kiwi fruit, apple juice and lemon juice in a blender and whizz until smooth. Stir in the orange rind. Pour the mixture into a 20cm/8in tray and freeze until almost firm. Spoon the frozen mixture into a mixing bowl, and beat until fluffy. Return the mixture to the tray, and freeze again until firm. Leave out at room temperature for about 10 minutes before serving.

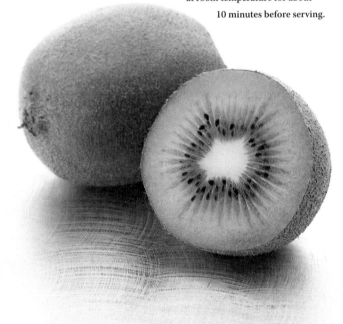

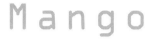

Mango

VITAMINS B3, C, E, BETA-CAROTENE; POTASSIUM; FIBRE

Regarded by many as the most delicious tropical fruit of all, mango offers many health benefits. It is perfect in fruit salads and desserts, but it works equally well in savoury dishes.

An average-sized mango contains almost the total recommended daily allowance of the antioxidant vitamin C, which produces collagen – a protein central to healthy skin and connective tissue. It also helps the body to heal faster from aches, pains, bumps and bruises.

Mango is one of the few fruit sources of vitamin E, an important antioxidant that helps to fight damaging free radicals in the body, as well as boosting the action of disease-battling antibodies and also speeding up post-exercise recovery rates. Together with vitamin C, the vitamin E in mango protects the brain from memory loss. With bright orange-yellow flesh, mangoes are high in beta-carotene, the precursor to antiviral vitamin A, which is needed for clear skin, healthy lungs, a strong heart and excellent overall immunity.

A powerful detoxifier, mango is a useful source of potassium, important for maintaining normal blood pressure. The fruit is full of fibre, which is vital for a well-functioning digestive system.

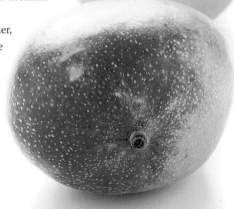

MANGO SMOOTHIE *serves 2*

1 mango, peeled, pitted and sliced
½ pineapple, peeled, cored and chopped
10 strawberries, hulled
80ml/2½fl oz/⅓ cup pineapple juice
75g/2½oz/⅓ cup plain
  bio-yogurt

**Place all the ingredients in a blender
and whizz until smooth and creamy.
Serve immediately.**

MANGO LASSI

500g/1lb 2oz/2 cups plain bio-yogurt
1½ mangoes, peeled, pitted and sliced
55g/2oz/¼ cup caster sugar
8 ice cubes
4 pistachios
4 almonds
a pinch of saffron threads

**Blend the yogurt, mango, sugar and
ice until frothy. Cut the pistachios
and almonds into slivers. Pour the
lassi into glasses and garnish with
the nuts and saffron threads.**

TROPICAL FRUIT SALAD

1 mango, peeled, pitted and cubed
4 kiwi fruits, peeled and sliced
1 papaya, peeled, deseeded and sliced
8 lychees, peeled, stoned and halved
1 pineapple, peeled, cored and cubed
pulp of 4 passion fruit

**Combine all the ingredients together
in a large bowl. Leave for an hour for
the juices to mingle, then serve.**

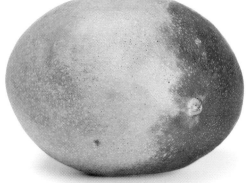

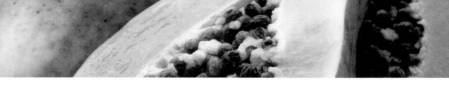

Papaya

VITAMINS B3, B5, C, BETA-CAROTENE, BIOTIN, FOLIC ACID; CALCIUM, IODINE,
IRON, MAGNESIUM, MANGANESE, PHOSPHORUS, POTASSIUM, SELENIUM, ZINC;
PAPAIN, FIBRE; CARBOHYDRATE

**First used in Mayan medicine, papayas have beautiful
yellow-orange flesh and are packed with carotenoids,
helpful for many diseases. Also known as paw paw,
papaya can be eaten ripe as a succulent fresh fruit or
cooked in curries and stews in its unripe green state.**

Papaya comes out on top in the antioxidant stakes, with half an average
fruit providing a whopping 38 milligrams of powerful carotenoids. It can
thus help to protect against cancer and cardiovascular disease, and to
treat skin irritations. Papaya contains protease enzymes, such as papain,
which are similar to those present in the stomach, therefore favouring
healthy digestion. The enzymes also reduce inflammation in the body,
and so may be beneficial in easing joint pain from conditions such as
arthritis and sports injuries. Used topically, papain literally digests dead
skin cells and acts as a mild exfoliant. It is also
said to aid the healing of skin sores.

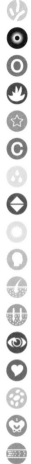

The fruit is a mild diuretic, and
is particularly useful in treating children's urinary and digestive ailments,
while its edible seeds have been used to
treat stomach aches and fungal infections.
Papaya is an excellent source of vitamin C.
As well as supporting the immune
system, this antioxidant prevents the build-up of plaque
in blood-vessels. Papaya is
rich in fibre, which low-
ers cholesterol levels
and helps to prevent
colon cancer by bind-
ing with toxins.

*PAPAYA EXFOLIATING LOTION
to brighten and rejuvenate the skin

1 large fresh papaya
piece of muslin
1 cup chamomile infusion, cooled

Peel the papaya, remove the seeds and purée the flesh in a blender. Press the purée through a piece of muslin to extract all the juice. Mix the juice with an equal amount of chamomile infusion, and stir well. Using cotton wool balls, apply the lotion to the face and neck, avoiding contact with the eyes. Leave for about 10 minutes, then rinse off. Keeps in the fridge for up to 2 days.

THAI-STYLE SALAD

2 papayas, peeled and deseeded
1 red pepper, deseeded
8 spring onions, trimmed and chopped
100g/3½oz/2 cups beansprouts
1 large handful mint, chopped
1 tbsp sugar
1 tbsp lime juice
1 tbsp fish sauce

Dice the papaya and the red pepper into 1cm/½in cubes. Toss all the ingredients in a large bowl, mixing well, and serve.

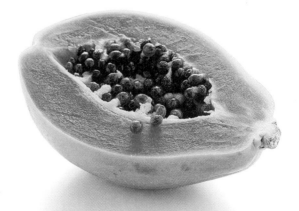

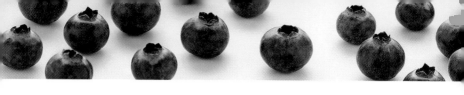

Blueberry

VITAMINS B2, B3, B5, C, E, K, BETA-CAROTENE, FOLIC ACID; CALCIUM, IRON, MAGNESIUM, MANGANESE, PHOSPHORUS, POTASSIUM, SELENIUM, ZINC; FLAVONOIDS, ELLAGIC ACID, TANNINS; FIBRE, CARBOHYDRATE

Blueberries are the number one fruit for helping to protect cells from free radical damage and aging, containing great youth-preserving antioxidants, which boost immunity and stave off many conditions. Historically a resource for herbalists and physicians, this sometimes tart, scented fruit prevents the growth of "unfriendly" bacteria to keep the gut clean and healthy.

According to research, one average serving of blueberries provides as many antioxidants as five average servings of broccoli, apples or carrots, and this superfood ranks top in antioxidant activity compared to 40 other fresh fruit and vegetables. Eat blueberries three or four times a week for full immunity-boosting benefits. They can be eaten raw as a snack, with plain bio-yogurt and nuts for a light breakfast, or combined with other berries and a little cream for a delicious dessert.

The berries get their beautiful blue colour from anthocyanins – potent antioxidants that combat cell damage, improve circulation and help to protect against heart problems, stroke, cancer and gum disease, and to enhance eyesight. Ellagic acid, another antioxidant found in blueberries, and the compound resveratrol, are also thought to help to prevent the development of cancer.

The proanthocyanidins (a type of flavonoids) contained in blueberries increase the potency of its vitamin-C content, so supporting collagen, which helps to keep the skin elastic. They also protect the eyes and blood vessels. Another useful compound in blueberries is pterostilbene, which has anti-diabetic and cholesterol-lowering properties and may reduce cognitive decline.

Blueberries are a fine source of agents lethal to bacteria, especially *E.coli*, and are a common folk remedy for diarrhoea and stomach upsets. They are rich in tannins, which have an anti-inflammatory effect on the body's tissues, and are said to kill microbes and fight the bacteria that cause urinary tract infections. In addition they are a traditional remedy for the treatment of coughs and colds.

These "wonderberries" may also aid in the reversal of neurodegenerative symptoms, such as loss of balance and co-ordination. They help to improve brain function and have been found to protect against dementia, and to preserve memory and learning ability in old age.

Used topically, blueberries' fruit acid content helps them to act as a gentle astringent and peeling agent.

BLUEBERRY SMOOTHIE *serves 2–3*

250g/9oz/1⅔ cups blueberries
125g /4½oz/1 cup raspberries or
   other summer berries
125g/4oz/½ cup plain
   bio-yogurt

Whizz all the ingredients in a blender, then serve. When temperatures outside are sizzling, add four cubes of ice in the blender to make a cooling summer crush.

✦BLUEBERRY TEA *for coughs*

2 tbsp chopped blueberry leaves
250ml/9fl oz/1 cup water,
   just boiled
clear honey, to taste

Place the leaves in the water. Leave to infuse for 5 minutes, then strain. Sweeten with honey to taste. Drink 1 cup every 4 hours.

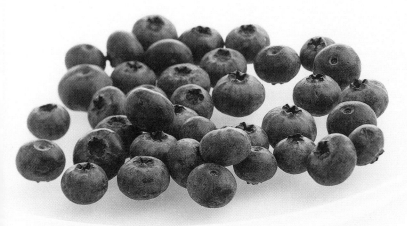

BLUEBERRY SAUCE

250g/9oz/1⅔ cups blueberries
80g/2¾oz/⅓ cup sugar
1 tbsp lemon juice
a pinch of salt
½ tsp vanilla extract

Wash the blueberries and crush them in a bowl. Add the sugar, lemon juice and salt, and mix well. In a saucepan heat the mixture and boil for 1 minute, then add the vanilla extract. Serve with puddings, cake or ice cream. Keeps in the fridge for 5 days.

BLUEBERRY AND PEAR CRUMBLE

85g/3oz butter, diced
85g/3oz/¾ cup plain flour
40g/1½oz/½ cup porridge oats
4 tbsp brown sugar
2 large pears, cored and sliced
80g/2¾oz/½ cup blueberries

Preheat the oven to 180°C/350°F/gas mark 4. Rub the butter into the flour in a mixing bowl until the mixture is like breadcrumbs. Stir in the porridge oats and brown sugar. Mix together the pears and blueberries in a greased baking dish. Sprinkle the crumble mixture over the top and cook for 40–45 minutes until browned on top.

BLUEBERRY FOOL

500g/1lb 2oz silken tofu
200ml/7fl oz/¾ cup apple juice
250g/9oz/1⅔ cups blueberries,
    plus extra to serve
300ml/10½fl oz/1¼ cups agave syrup
100ml/3½fl oz/⅓ cup unrefined
    sunflower oil
1 tsp vanilla extract

Put the tofu and apple juice in a food processor and whizz until smooth. Add the remaining ingredients and continue to blend until thick and creamy. Spoon into dessert glasses and serve chilled, decorated with a few blueberries on the top.

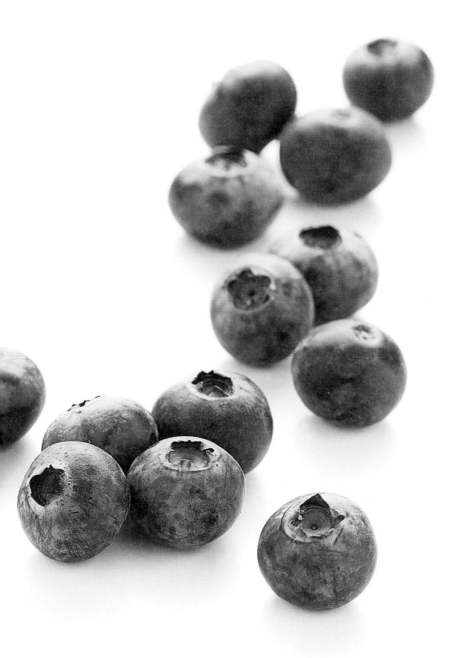

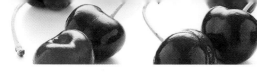

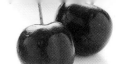

Cherry

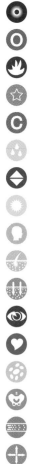

VITAMINS B3, B5, C; BETA-CAROTENE, BIOTIN, FOLIC ACID; BORON, CALCIUM, IRON, MAGNESIUM, MANGANESE, PHOSPHORUS, POTASSIUM, SELENIUM; QUERCETIN, FLAVONOIDS, ELLAGIC ACID; FIBRE; CARBOHYDRATE

These sweet summer treats are potent detoxifiers and are packed with antioxidants, making them excellent immunity boosters.

Cherries are rich in flavonoids such as anthocyanins, antioxidant substances that the body uses to help to make disease-fighting chemicals. Aching joints and fragile bones are an unwelcome symptom of aging, but cherries can do a lot to protect them. They supply the mineral boron, which may help to prevent the steady loss of bone density with advancing age. And their rich anthocyanin content acts as a powerful anti-inflammatory, combating pain in joints and muscles, as well as fibromyalgia – pain in the fibrous tissues of the body, such as the muscles, tendons and ligaments. These antioxidants can also strengthen blood vessels and slow down the aging process of the skin. And it is also the anthocyanins in cherries that give them the same heart-protective effects as red wine. These benefits in turn help people to stay active, which promotes general good health as well as better bone strength and increased physical coordination.

Cherries are a rich source of quercetin, another strong anti-inflammatory substance, which helps to relieve painful conditions such as rheumatoid arthritis, and gout – a form of arthritis that occurs when uric acid crystals accumulate in joints, leading to pain and inflammation. In studies, cherries have been found to significantly decrease uric acid levels, so limiting the formation of the gout-inducing crystals.

Like many other berries, cherries contain the phytochemical ellagic acid – a powerful compound that blocks an enzyme that cancer cells need in order to develop. They also contain selenium, a mineral with powerful immunity-boosting properties, and antioxidant vitamin C, which destroys free radicals in the body, aiding the fight against viruses and bacteria. In addition, vitamin C strengthens collagen, maintains healthy-looking skin and hair and helps to protect against eye disease.

Other antioxidants in cherries include superoxide dismutase (useful in joint, respiratory and gastrointestinal health) and melatonin – one of the most potent known free radical scavengers, which is important for the immune system. Low melatonin levels have been associated with sleep problems, so cherries could be useful to aid sleep. Melatonin is also commonly used to combat jetlag.

Cherry stalks can be made into an infusion that is a traditional remedy for cystitis and bladder infections.

CHOCO-CHERRIES *serves 1–2*

200g/7oz/1 cup cherries, stalks left on
100g/3½oz good quality plain chocolate,
  melted

Dip each of the cherries into the chocolate. Place on a greased plate and chill until set.

CHERRY PARFAIT

300g/10½oz/1½ cups cherries, pitted
500g/1lb 2oz/2 cups plain bio-yogurt
  or soya yogurt
150g/5½oz crunchy granola cereal
2 tbsp desiccated coconut, plus extra
  to serve
1 tbsp cherry jam (optional)

Put all the ingredients in a food processor and blend until creamy. Serve chilled, sprinkled with extra coconut.

CHERRY AND RHUBARB COMPÔTE

400g/14oz/2 cups cherries, pitted
3 rhubarb stalks, chopped
3 tbsp apple juice
2 tbsp fruit sugar
plain bio-yogurt, to serve

Put all the ingredients in a saucepan. Bring to the boil, reduce the heat and simmer, covered, for 8 minutes, stirring occasionally. Serve with plain bio-yogurt.

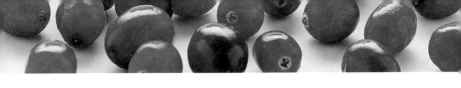

Cranberry
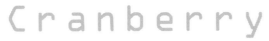

VITAMINS B5, C, K, BETA-CAROTENE, FOLIC ACID; CALCIUM, IRON, MAGNESIUM, MANGANESE; PHOSPHORUS, POTASSIUM, SELENIUM; ELLAGIC ACID, FLAVONOIDS, TANNINS; FIBRE; CARBOHYDRATE

These tart, tangy berries are high in antioxidant vitamin C, making them great immunity-boosters.

Native North Americans first introduced Europeans to cranberries to help them to combat scurvy, and it became recognized that the acidity of cranberries increases the natural acidity of urine, thus preventing bacteria from thriving. One of the natural-health success stories of the past few years, cranberries have proved their value in preventing urinary tract infections, such as cystitis. The powerful ingredient is a flavonoid called proanthocyanidins, which is more abundant in cranberries than in most other fruits. Proanthocyanidins prevent bacteria sticking to the urinary tract wall, and prevent infections of the stomach in the same way. Other compounds in this berry have been found to inhibit plaque-causing bacteria in the mouth, which causes tooth decay and gum disease. Cranberries can also combat kidney stone formation.

A valuable source of antioxidant vitamin C, cranberries are also rich in beta-carotene and folic acid, enabling them to help to ward off colds, flu and many other diseases, including some cancers. Many people now eat cranberries every day, as a first line of defence.

If you have difficulty finding the fresh berries, buy dried cranberries, juice or extract instead. For maximum benefit, drink a glass of unsweetened cranberry juice or take 800mg of cranberry extract daily.

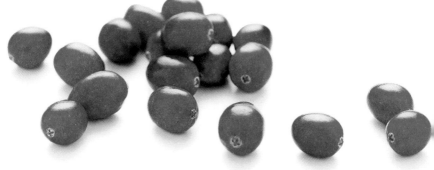

CRANBERRY AND BANANA SMOOTHIE

300ml/10½fl oz/1¼ cups unsweetened
 cranberry juice
350ml/10½fl oz/1¼ cups white grape juice
2 bananas, chopped
10 strawberries, hulled
400g/14oz/1⅔ cups plain bio-yogurt or
 soya yogurt
3 tbsp clear honey

Put all the ingredients in a blender and whizz until smooth. Drink immediately.

CRANBERRY-ORANGE RELISH

300g/12oz/2 cups cranberries, fresh
 or frozen
1 orange, unpeeled, cut into eighths and
 deseeded
1 apple, unpeeled, cut into eighths and
 cored
75g/2½oz/⅓ cup sugar
1 tsp ground ginger

Blend the fruit in a food processor. Stir in the sugar and ginger, and transfer to a glass jar. Cover with a lid and refrigerate for at least 4 hours. Use when needed.

CRANBERRY SAUCE

115g/4oz/½ cup dried cranberries
250ml/9fl oz/1 cup cranberry
 or orange juice
2.5cm/1in piece root ginger, peeled and
 finely chopped
1 tbsp red wine (optional)
2 tbsp clear honey

Place the cranberries and juice in a pan and soak for 30 minutes. Bring to the boil, add the ginger and wine, if using, reduce the heat and simmer for 10 minutes, stirring. Mix in the honey and serve with meat or a nut roast.

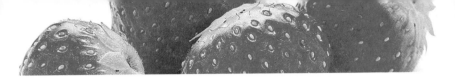

Strawberry

Vitamins B2, B3, B5, B6, C, K, folic acid; copper, iron, magnesium, manganese, iodine, potassium; flavonoids; fibre; omega-3 fatty acids; ellagic acid

These favourite berries have been popular throughout the ages and were prized for their therapeutic properties in ancient Rome. Strawberries enhance liver and gallbladder functions, and are a traditional remedy for treating gout, arthritis and kidney stones.

One of the delights of summer, strawberries are full of disease-fighting and age-defying nutrients. Packed with vitamin C, an average serving of strawberries gives twice the recommended daily adult intake of this immunity-boosting vitamin. Try fresh strawberries with a pinch of pepper for a novel taste with a sharp edge. The vitamin C in strawberries is essential for the manufacture of collagen – a protein that helps to maintain the structure of the skin, keeping it elastic and young-looking. Vitamin C also plays an important role in healing wounds and can ward off gingivitis, the gum disease that affects three out of four adults. It can also help to dissolve tartarous incrustations on the teeth.

Strawberries contain ellagic acid, a phytochemical shown to help fight cancer and destroy some of the toxins in cigarette smoke and polluted air. Their B-vitamin content makes them useful for supporting the nervous system and fighting stress-related conditions, as well as building resistance to disease, while their high iron content makes them therapeutic for anaemia and fatigue.

The berries are rich in fibre for a healthy heart and digestive system. Strawberries also have a mild laxative effect and may help to regenerate intestinal flora.

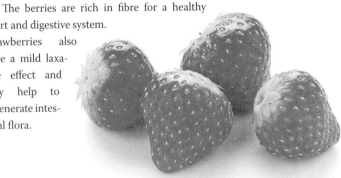

STRAWBERRY AND RICOTTA SPREAD

150g/5½oz/1 cup strawberries, hulled

2 limes

2 tsp icing sugar

100g/3oz/scant ½ cup ricotta cheese

cinnamon bagels, to serve

Mash the strawberries with a fork and grate the zest of the limes. Add the icing sugar and the lime zest and stir well into the ricotta cheese to form a smooth mixture. Spread over toasted cinnamon bagels for a delicious breakfast treat.

STRAWBERRY SMOOTHIE *serves 2*

150g/5½oz/1 cup strawberries, hulled

1 banana, chopped

1 small pot plain bio-yogurt

150ml/5fl oz/scant ⅔ cup unsweetened
 soya milk

mint leaves, to decorate

Place all the ingredients in a blender and whizz until smooth. Serve in tall glasses topped with mint leaves.

GRILLED FRUIT KEBABS

3 kiwi fruit, peeled

½ pineapple, peeled and cored

3 bananas

16 strawberries

6 tbsp pineapple juice

2 tbsp agave syrup or clear honey

Cut the kiwis, pineapple and bananas into 2.5cm/1in cubes. Thread alternate pieces of the cut-up fruit and strawberries onto wooden skewers. Combine the pineapple juice and agave syrup or honey in a bowl and use it to brush the kebabs. Then, place them under a grill for about 6 minutes, turning frequently.

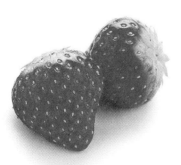

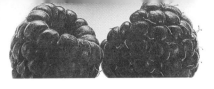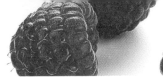

Raspberry

VITAMINS B2, B3, B5, C, E, K, BETA-CAROTENE, BIOTIN, FOLIC ACID; CALCIUM, COPPER, IODINE, IRON, MAGNESIUM, MANGANESE, PHOSPHORUS, POTASSIUM, SELENIUM, ZINC; ELLAGIC ACID; FLAVONOIDS; FIBRE

These jewel-like, soft berries are packed with health-enhancing antioxidants and other protective nutrients that are powerful fighters of infections and diseases, including cancer and heart problems.

One of the top fruit sources of fibre, raspberries are helpful for keeping cholesterol low and improving digestion, as well as detoxifying the body and keeping blood-sugar levels steady. Raspberries are naturally astringent and can therefore help to treat upset stomachs and diarrhoea. They have antimicrobial effects that can prevent the proliferation of bacteria and fungi in the digestive system. One of these, *Candida albicans*, causes the irritating vaginal infection called thrush and has also been linked with digestive disorders such as irritable bowel syndrome. Raspberries are also said to protect against allergies.

Like other berries, raspberries are high in anthocyanins, powerful antioxidants that help the body to produce cells to fight off unwanted invaders. The anthocyanins in raspberries have anti-inflammatory properties, thus protecting from conditions such as arthritis.

The fruits also contain ellagic acid, which is anti-carcinogenic and prevents adverse cellular changes and may be especially useful for preventing cancers of the mouth, throat and colon. It is also thought to promote the healing of wounds.

Raspberries contain high levels of infection-fighting vitamin C, which boosts immunity and can help to prevent everything from heart disease to eye problems. They are packed with a host of absorbable minerals, including calcium, potassium, iron and magnesium, all of which are essential to general good health. Raspberries are also particularly helpful to those suffering from heart problems, fatigue and depression, as well as convalescents.

Traditionally, an infusion made from raspberry leaves can facilitate labour by acting as a uterine relaxant and a tonic.

RASPBERRY BRULÉE

400g/14oz/3¼ cups raspberries
1 tsp vanilla extract
300g/10½oz/scant 1¼ cups plain
  bio-yogurt
6 tsp sugar

Place the raspberries in 4 ramekins or small dishes. Combine the vanilla extract and yogurt, and spoon the mixture over the fruit. Cover the surface of each ramekin with the sugar, then caramelize under a very hot grill for 2 minutes, or until crisp. Allow to cool, then serve.

RASPBERRY COULIS

450g/1lb/3½ cups raspberries
1 tbsp fruit sugar
1 tsp lemon juice

Put all the ingredients in a food processor and blend. Pour the mixture through a fine sieve into a bowl, pressing on the solids. Serve the sauce on top of ice-cream or other desserts.

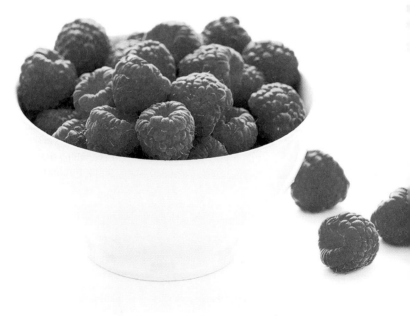

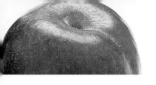
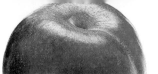
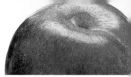

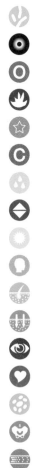

Plum and prune

VITAMINS A, B2, B3, B5, B6, C, BETA-CAROTENE, FOLIC ACID; CALCIUM, COPPER, IODINE, IRON, MAGNESIUM, MANGANESE, PHOSPHORUS, POTASSIUM, SELENIUM, ZINC; MALIC ACD; CARBOHYDRATE; FIBRE

This versatile fruit can be eaten fresh or dried and is a useful source of immunity-boosting antioxidants

Plums are rich in pectin, a type of soluble fibre that absorbs and neutralizes toxins in the large intestine, which means that they have excellent detoxifying properties. They're great for helping anyone who is prone to anaemia because they're packed with iron, which is crucial in the formation of red blood cells. They also contain malic acid and the antioxidant vitamin C, which enhance the absorption of iron.

Prunes are dried plums, both of which have made headlines in relation to their rich phytochemical content, namely neochlorogenic and chlorogenic acids. These antioxidant compounds help to neutralize hazardous free radicals in the body, protecting cells from damage and slowing down the aging process.

Containing many of the same nutrients as fresh plums, prunes also have a very beneficial effect on the digestive system. They have long been used as the most effective, yet gentle, natural remedy for constipation. Prunes contain a natural laxative called diphenylisatin, which is why they are so useful for keeping the bowel regular. Their fibre-rich bulk softens food waste that has dried out during an excessive delay in the colon, and helps it move painlessly on and out of the body. Yet they may also slow the movement of food from the stomach if it is emptying too quickly, causing indigestion or wind. Prunes are known to lower cholesterol by helping the body to excrete fats, and feeding the good bacteria in the intestine, helping to prevent harmful bacteria breeding.

While prunes have long been regarded as a rich source of fibre, it is perhaps less well-known that, weight for weight, they are the most potent of all antioxidant foods. Eating prunes is also a sweet way of increasing beta-carotene and potassium intake. Their high level of potassium keeps blood pressure in check, while their vitamin B6 protects the heart and boosts brain power. Like plums, prunes are also full of iron, which provides energy and prevents fatigue, making them an ideal snack for anyone who exercises strenuously. Their combination of iron and vitamin A is especially good for stimulating hair growth, while vitamin A itself maintains youthful skin and protects the eyes.

AROMATIC STEWED PRUNES *serves 2*

250g/9oz/scant 1 cup soft pitted prunes
juice of 2 oranges
a pinch of ground cinnamon
plain bio-yogurt, to serve

Put the prunes in a pan with the orange juice and cinnamon, and bring to the boil. Reduce the heat, then simmer, covered, for about 15 minutes. Serve with yogurt.

PLUM COMPÔTE *serves 2*

16 ripe but firm plums
2 tsp ground allspice
2 tbsp dark brown sugar
250ml/9fl oz/1 cup orange juice
grated zest of ½ orange
plain bio-yogurt, to serve

Place the plums in a large ovenproof dish. Add the allspice, sugar, orange juice and zest, and bake in a preheated oven at 180°C/350°F/ gas mark 4 for 30 minutes. Serve with the yogurt.

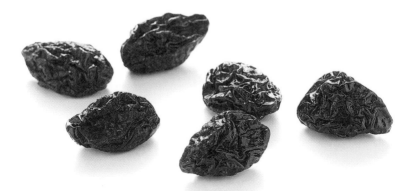

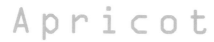

Apricot

VITAMINS A, B2, B3, B5, C; BETA-CAROTENE, LYCOPENE; CALCIUM, IRON, POTASSIUM; ZINC; FIBRE; TRYPTOPHAN

As their bright orange colour shows, apricots are rich in beta-carotene. They have been prominent in Indian and Chinese folklore for 2,000 years. These fragrant stone fruits are bursting with nutrients, and are delicious eaten fresh or dried.

Apricots are thought to have originated in ancient Armenia, although they have a long history throughout Asia and the near East.

These flavoursome fruits have high levels of beta-carotene, which the body turns into antiviral and anti-carcinogenic vitamin A. It is the most abundant antioxidant found in apricots, helping to protect the skin and lungs from oxidation damage and supporting the immune system. It also prevents free radicals from damaging the eyes. Eating fresh apricots can be helpful to those suffering from infections, particularly those of the respiratory tract. Dried apricots supply iron and produce haemoglobin, which is beneficial to those suffering from anaemia. They also have a balancing effect on the nervous system, treating mental fatigue, mild anxiety and insomnia, and yield an oil that is highly nourishing for the skin.

Apricots are an excellent source of vitamin B5, which is crucial for the production of anti-bodies. They are also high in vitamin C, which is essential for all immune functions. In addition, apricots contain lycopene, which is one of the most powerful antioxidants. Lycopene is known for its ability to prevent the build-up of fatty deposits in the arteries and it also has strong anti-carcinogenic properties.

Apricots are rich in the amino acid tryptophan, which the body converts to the feel-good chemical serotonin. This brain chemical lifts your mood, making you feel more optimistic, improving self-esteem and even helping to control impulsive behaviour. And it helps you sleep well too. Some of the tryptophan is also converted to niacin, or vitamin B3, if necessary. A shortage of this nutrient can cause lethargy, so eating apricots can keep energy levels high.

APRICOT CRUMBLE

950g/2lb 2oz apricots, peeled, halved,
  pitted and roughly chopped
70g/2½oz/⅓ cup sugar
100g/3½oz/⅔ cup wholemeal flour
25g/1oz/¼ cup oats
2 tbsp demerara sugar
55g/2oz unsalted butter, cut into
  small pieces
crème fraîche, to serve (optional)

Preheat the oven to 190°C/ 375°F/gas mark 5. Place the apricots in a baking dish. Sprinkle over 55g/2oz/¼ cup of the sugar. In another bowl, combine the remaining ingredients and rub together until the mixture resembles breadcrumbs. Cover the apricots with the crumble and cook for 40 minutes. Serve with crème fraîche, if desired.

*APRICOT MASSAGE OIL
for dry, sensitive skins

250g/9oz apricot seeds
750ml/26fl oz/3 cups carrier (base) oil,
  such as almond or olive
piece of muslin

With a pestle and mortar, grind the seeds to release the oils, then place them in a clear glass jar. Pour the carrier oil onto the seeds, secure and shake. Place in a sunny spot and leave for 2 to 6 weeks. Pour the oil through a muslin-lined sieve into a jug, then pour into dark glass bottles. Store for up to a year. Apply liberally to the skin when needed.

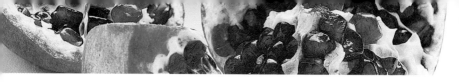

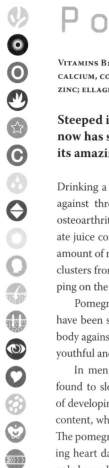

Pomegranate
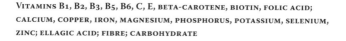

VITAMINS B1, B2, B3, B5, B6, C, E, BETA-CAROTENE, BIOTIN, FOLIC ACID;
CALCIUM, COPPER, IRON, MAGNESIUM, PHOSPHORUS, POTASSIUM, SELENIUM,
ZINC; ELLAGIC ACID; FIBRE; CARBOHYDRATE

Steeped in symbolism since ancient times, pomegranate now has superfood status, thanks to recent research into its amazing healing attributes.

Drinking a glass of pomegranate juice a day could help to protect you against three major problems of old age: heart disease, cancer and osteoarthritis. According to studies, a medium-sized glass of pomegranate juice contains almost three times as many antioxidants as the same amount of red wine, green tea or orange juice. Removing the edible seed clusters from the fruit can seem tricky, but you can do this easily by tapping on the outside with a wooden spoon until they fall out.

Pomegranate is abundant in antioxidants called punicalagins, which have been shown to prevent several forms of cancer by protecting the body against free radicals, which can harm cells. They also keep the skin youthful and protect it from sun damage.

In men who already have prostate cancer, pomegranate has been found to slow the rate of tumour growth. It may also reduce the risk of developing various cancers because of its extremely high ellagic acid content, which has anti-carcinogenic and anti-heart disease properties. The pomegranate's polyphenols work as powerful antioxidants, preventing heart damage and the build-up of plaque in the arteries. They not only lower high blood pressure but also help to fight LDL "bad" cholesterol, which is linked to heart attacks and strokes.

Pomegranate eases the pain and disability of osteoarthritis by slowing the deterioration of cartilage and preventing inflammation. It contains plenty of healing vitamins including B1, which helps the body to convert food into energy, and B2, which helps to tame free radicals and is also central to memory function. Its vitamin C content also offers protection against cardiovascular disease, cancer and eye problems. Pomegranate may also have antiviral and anti-bacterial properties, and has been shown to discourage the formation of dental plaque.

FRUIT SALAD WITH POMEGRANATE

1 pomegranate
1 bunch white seedless grapes, destalked
150g/5½oz/1 cup strawberries, hulled
   and chopped
1 banana, chopped
1 peach, pitted and chopped
100g/3½oz/⅔ cup blueberries
4 tbsp fruit juice of choice
1 tbsp lemon juice
1 tbsp clear honey
a pinch of ground nutmeg, to serve

Cut the pomegranate in half horizontally and, using a wooden spoon, bash until the seeds fall out. Put them in a bowl with the other fruit. Combine the fruit juice, lemon juice and honey, pour it over the fruit and mix gently. Serve sprinkled with the nutmeg.

POMEGRANATE CUP

200g/7oz/¾ cup plain bio-yogurt
2 tsp clear honey
4 pomegranates
4 mint sprigs, to serve

Place the yogurt in a small bowl and stir in the honey until well combined. Cut each pomegranate in half horizontally and, using a wooden spoon, bash until the seeds fall out. Mix the pomegranate seeds with the yogurt and honey mixture, garnish with mint, and serve.

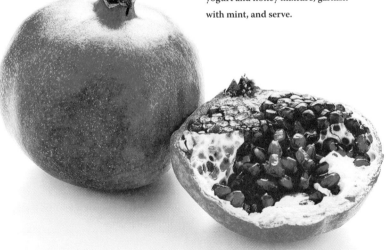

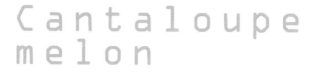

Cantaloupe melon

VITAMINS A, B3, B6, C, BETA-CAROTENE, FOLIC ACID; POTASSIUM; FIBRE

These succulent summer fruits offer a mouth-watering slice of nutritional goodness bursting with antioxidants to fight aging free radicals.

Cantaloupe melon is also known as rock or musk melon. Just one average slice provides more beta-carotene and vitamin C than your body can use in a whole day. Cantaloupe melon is one of the richest sources of beta-carotene, which the body converts to vitamin A, an antioxidant that is crucial for the production of disease-fighting lymphocyte cells. This fruit is also rich in vitamin C, which we need for all immune functions and to protect us against colds, cancer and heart disease. Both vitamin C and beta-carotene are naturally anti-aging and aid cell repair and growth, as well as supporting the circulatory system.

Cantaloupe also contains potassium, which can lower high blood pressure and "bad" LDL cholesterol. Its high water content gives it a mildly diuretic action, helping to detoxify the body, while its B-vitamins enhance the production of energy and help to stabilize blood sugar.

The dense texture of this fragrant melon makes it a satisfying replacement for any foods you're limiting, just as their sweetness meets the need that might otherwise be filled by empty-calorie snacks.

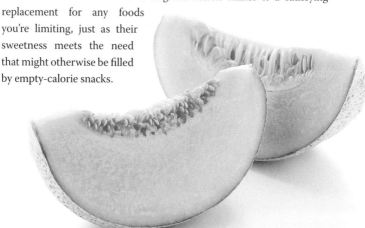

RED MELON SALAD

1 pink grapefruit, peeled

2 Cantaloupe melons, peeled, deseeded
    and cubed

10 raspberries

2.5cm/1in piece root ginger, peeled and
    grated

Divide the grapefruit into segments and combine with the melon in a large bowl. Leave for 30 minutes to allow the juices to mingle. Divide into four serving bowls and decorate with the raspberries and the ginger.

*MELON LOTION
to cool and hydrate the skin

¼ Cantaloupe melon

piece of muslin

½ lemon

1 tbsp olive oil

Whizz the melon in a blender, then filter the juice through the muslin. Squeeze the lemon to extract 1 teaspoon of juice. Combine the melon juice, lemon juice and olive oil in a container, cover and store in the fridge. Apply twice daily to the face and neck with cotton wool. Keeps in the fridge for up to 2 days.

MELON AND GINGER

2 small Canteloupe melons

2 tsp lime juice

2.5cm/1in piece root ginger,
    finely chopped

2 tsp ground cinnamon

4 tbsp cherries (optional)

Quarter the melons and cut away the skin. Scoop out and discard the seeds. Cut the flesh into wedges or scoop into balls. Add the lime juice and ginger and mix together well. Dust with cinnamon, top with cherries, if using, and serve.

Avocado

VITAMINS B1, B2, B3, B5, B6, C, E, K, BIOTIN, CAROTENOIDS, FOLIC ACID; CALCIUM, COPPER, IODINE, IRON, MAGNESIUM, MANGANESE, PHOSPHORUS, POTASSIUM, ZINC; BETA-SITOSTEROL, GLUTATHIONE; OMEGA-3, -6 AND -9 FATTY ACIDS; TRYPTOPHAN; LECITHIN; FIBRE

One of the few fruits that contains fat, avocado boasts a wealth of health-boosting properties

Strictly speaking, avocado is a type of pear and therefore a fruit, although it is typically used in savoury dishes. It is native to Central America, and was discovered by Spanish invaders in the sixteenth century. It is now popular throughout the world and grown in various tropical regions. With a smooth, buttery texture and mild, creamy taste, avocados are best eaten when ripe. As they are normally picked before they are ripe, avocados take about a week to ripen at room temperature, although storing them in a paper bag with a banana can speed the process.

Scientists have found that people are more relaxed after a higher-fat meal, and even feel less pain. No wonder people eat junk foods when they're feeling low! Avocados are the healthier alternative: instead of saturated fat, they provide healthy monounsaturated fat, which raises levels of "good" cholesterol while slightly lowering fatty triglycerides. Another type of fat in this delicious, creamy food is lecithin, which plays a role in improving brain function. Some fat is also necessary for the body to absorb nutrients that can improve your mood, such as avocado's vitamin E, which is also an antioxidant that neutralizes the damaging effect of toxins in the body, boosts resistance to infection and has an anti-aging effect.

The high content of vitamins C and E in avocados is excellent for keeping the skin soft, supple and healthy, and for maintaining glossy hair. They have high levels of the antioxidant lutein, which studies have shown helps to protect against eye problems and cardiovascular disease. Avocados are rich in tryptophan, along with vitamin B6 and folic acid, which help the body to turn tryptophan into the feel-good chemical serotonin. Just one avocado provides half the recommended daily intake of vitamin B6 – essential for helping the body to release energy from food. The folic acid promotes reproductive health.

Avocados are rich in potassium, which staves off fatigue, depression, heart disease and strokes and is essential for healthy blood pressure and muscle contraction. They are said to have a unique anti-bacterial and anti-fungal substance in the pulp, as well as to harmonizing the liver and soothing the nervous system.

Loaded with fibre, avocados are also a source of linoleic acid (known as omega-6 fatty acid), which the body converts to gamma-linolenic acid (GLA), a substance that helps to thin the blood, soothe inflammation and improve blood-sugar balance. They are high in omega-3 fatty acids, so helping to prevent wrinkles, enhance brain power and treat arthritis. They also contain oleic acid, the building block for omega-9 fatty acids, which are excellent for the skin and have anti-inflammatory properties.

Avocado's range of B-vitamins help the immune cells to destroy harmful invaders – as does glutathione, a powerful substance that boosts the action of the body's natural killer cells. In addition, they contain the plant chemical beta-sitosterol, which lowers "bad" cholesterol and is particularly beneficial to the prostate gland.

Shunned by dieters because of their high calorie count, avocados may aid weight loss by satisfying hunger and improving metabolism. With 20 vitamins, minerals and phytonutrients, avocados are one of nature's true superfoods for anyone aiming to get fit. They contain more protein than any other fruit, making them great for strength and endurance.

✳ AVOCADO FACE PACK *to rejuvenate tired skin*

1 avocado, pitted and peeled	**Combine all the ingredients in a bowl**
1 tsp clear honey	**and mash into a paste. Leave in the**
1 tsp lemon juice	**fridge for 30 minutes. Apply the pack**
1 tsp plain yogurt	**to your face and leave for 10 minutes**
	before removing with cool water.

AVOCADO AND BABY SPINACH SALAD

juice of 2 limes

2 tsp clear honey

a pinch of salt

2 avocados, pitted, peeled and cubed

16 cherry tomatoes, halved

2 handfuls baby spinach, washed and torn
   into pieces

Make the dressing by combining
the lime juice, honey and salt in
a jug, and shaking well. Put all
the remaining ingredients in
a bowl and coat with the dressing.
Mix gently and serve immediately.

GUACAMOLE *makes 1 large bowl*

2 avocados, pitted and peeled

juice of 1 lime

2 garlic cloves, crushed

1 onion, finely chopped

2 tomatoes, skinned and chopped

1 small red chilli, deseeded and finely
   chopped

1 tbsp coriander, finely chopped

For a chunky dip, mash the avocados
by hand with the lime juice until
smooth, then add the remaining
ingredients and combine thoroughly.
For a smoother texture, blend the
ingredients in a food processor.
Serve as a dip for crudités.

TANGY SUMMER SALAD

3 tbsp olive oil

1 tsp clear honey

1 red onion, grated

1 tsp Dijon mustard

4 avocados, pitted, peeled and sliced

1 pink grapefruit, peeled and broken into
   segments

1 large handful rocket leaves

Whisk the oil, honey, onion and
mustard together in a bowl. Add the
avocados, grapefruit and rocket, toss
well in the dressing and serve.

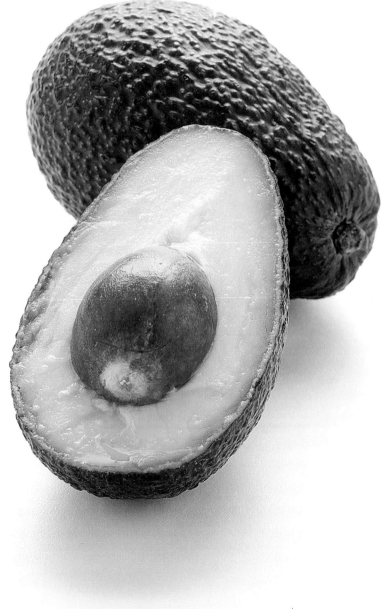

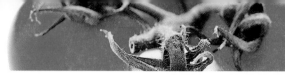

Tomato

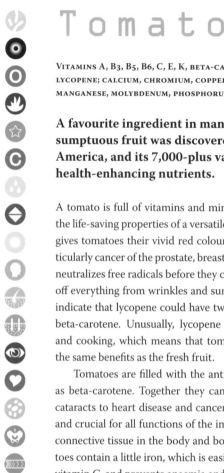

Vitamins A, B3, B5, B6, C, E, K, beta-carotene, biotin, folic acid, lycopene; calcium, chromium, copper, iodine, iron, magnesium, manganese, molybdenum, phosphorus, potassium, zinc; fibre

A favourite ingredient in many dishes, this juicy, sumptuous fruit was discovered by the Aztecs of Central America, and its 7,000-plus varieties are all packed with health-enhancing nutrients.

A tomato is full of vitamins and minerals, but it is most renowned for the life-saving properties of a versatile caretenoid called lycopene, which gives tomatoes their vivid red colour and helps to prevent cancer, particularly cancer of the prostate, breast, lung and endometrium. Lycopene neutralizes free radicals before they can cause damage, therefore staving off everything from wrinkles and sun-damage to heart attacks. Studies indicate that lycopene could have twice the anti-carcinogenic punch of beta-carotene. Unusually, lycopene is unharmed by food processing and cooking, which means that tomato-based products offer many of the same benefits as the fresh fruit.

Tomatoes are filled with the antioxidant vitamins C and E, as well as beta-carotene. Together they can help to prevent everything from cataracts to heart disease and cancer. Vitamin C is powerfully antiviral and crucial for all functions of the immune system and it also supports connective tissue in the body and boosts immunity. In addition, tomatoes contain a little iron, which is easily absorbed when accompanied by vitamin C, and prevents anaemia and fatigue.

The high levels of beta-carotene in tomatoes are necessary for the production of vitamin A. This helps to maintain a healthy thymus gland, which plays a vital role in immune response. Tomatoes are also rich in potassium, which regulates fluid balance.

A bottle of tomato juice keeps minerals at a safe level when you're running. Most of us get too much sodium in our diet, but a long run can dangerously reduce the body's levels of minerals, particularly sodium – especially if you've drunk a lot of water. A drink of bought tomato juice replenishes fluid and sodium.

GAZPACHO

6 ripe tomatoes, chopped
½ onion, finely chopped
½ cucumber, peeled and diced
1 green pepper, deseeded and diced
juice of 1 lemon
3 garlic cloves, chopped
3 tbsp chopped parsley
2 tsp vegetable stock powder

Place all the ingredients in a blender and whizz until smooth. Divide into four bowls. Chill for 30 minutes, then serve.

SUN-DRIED TOMATO PESTO

24 sun-dried tomatoes in oil
80g/2¾oz/½ cup macadamia nuts, chopped
150g/5oz basil
3 garlic cloves, crushed
1½ tsp tomato purée
1 tbsp balsamic vinegar
1 tbsp lemon juice
250ml/9fl oz/1 cup tomato juice
4 tbsp olive oil
salt and ground black pepper

Blend all the ingredients together in a food processor until smooth. Transfer to a bowl and season to taste. Store for up to 5 days in the fridge.

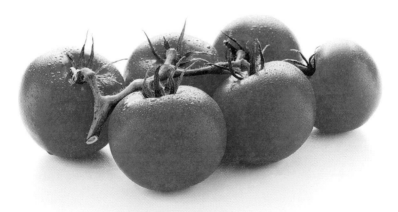

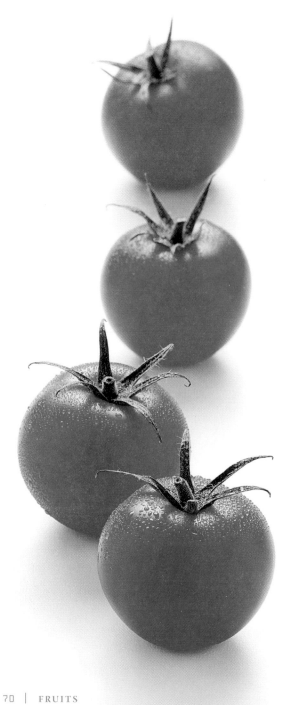

SPICY GARDEN COCKTAIL

4 tomatoes

4 small cucumbers

8 celery stalks, with leaves

celery salt, optional

hot chilli sauce, to taste

ice cubes

Cut the tomatoes into chunks and the cucumbers into strips. Remove the celery tops from the stalks, reserving 4 to garnish. Feed the tomatoes, cucumbers and celery stalks through a juicer. Coat the rims of 4 tall glasses with celery salt, if using, and pour the juice into the glasses. Add the chilli sauce to taste and several ice cubes. Stir well. Garnish with the celery tops and serve immediately.

CHILLED TOMATO SOUP

8 tomatoes, skinned, deseeded and
    chopped

2 cucumbers, diced

1 l/35fl oz/4 cups tomato juice

2 sweet peppers, deseeded
    and diced

2 garlic cloves, crushed

1 tbsp red wine vinegar

1 tbsp olive oil

Blend half the tomatoes, half the cucumbers, the juice, sweet peppers, garlic and vinegar in a blender. Stir in the oil and remaining tomatoes and cucumber. Chill for 30 minutes before serving.

TOMATO RAITA

30 cherry tomatoes

400g/14oz/1⅔ cups plain bio-yogurt

1 spring onion, trimmed and finely
    chopped

1 tbsp finely chopped coriander

1 tbsp finely chopped mint

½ tsp roasted ground cumin

salt, to taste

Cut the tomatoes into quarters, place them in an ovenproof dish and grill until slightly soft. Leave to cool, then transfer to a bowl. Add the yogurt, spring onion, coriander, mint, cumin and salt. Mix well and serve as a dip.

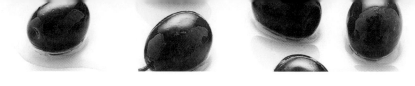

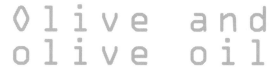

Olive and olive oil

Vitamins E, K, beta-carotene; calcium, copper, iodine, iron, magnesium, manganese, phosphorus, potassium, selenium, zinc; polyphenols; omega-9 fatty acids; fibre

The regular consumption of olives and olive oil in Mediterranean countries could explain the robust health enjoyed by many people who live there.

There are hundreds of olive varieties. In general, black varieties are moist and full flavoured, while green have a milder taste. One recent scientific study suggests that eating olives on a regular basis can play an important role in protecting bones against osteoporosis and is associated with a lower risk of colon cancer, which becomes more common in later age.

Olives also contain a substance called squalene, which has heart-protecting properties, and the phytochemicals oleoeuropein, which lowers high blood pressure, and oleocanthal, which relieves inflammation.

Olive oil is a monounsaturated fat that is believed to have anti-carcinogenic properties, and helps to lower high blood pressure and prevent diabetes. It lowers levels of harmful LDL cholesterol while leaving the beneficial HDL cholesterol alone. Research into the effectiveness of olive oil against clogging of the arteries reveals that the olives' monounsaturated fats prevent the oxidation of cholesterol, and therefore stop it from sticking to artery walls and causing heart attacks.

Further studies suggest that olive oil also contains hefty concentrations of antioxidants, including chlorophyll, carotenoids and polyphenolic compounds – all of which not only fight age-accelerating free radicals, but also protect the olives' important vitamin E content. Their rich supply of polyphenols, known to have anti-inflammatory and anticoagulant actions, are also thought to help stave off conditions such as osteoporosis and arthritis.

Olive oil is high in oleic acid, an omega-9 fatty acid, which demonstrates anti-inflammatory properties to calm and soothe the skin. In addition, the essential fatty acids in olives have been shown to boost the body's ability to remove unwanted stored fat in the cells. Rich in vitamin E, which helps to keep skin wrinkle-free and hair glossy, it also stimulates the secretion of bile, helping to soften and expel gallstones. The vitamin E content can also reduce the severity of hot flushes.

Used topically, olive oil makes an excellent skin moisturizer and hair conditioner, and can also soften wax inside the ears.

TAPENADE

200g/7oz/scant 1¼ cups olives, pitted and chopped
55g/2oz capers, drained and chopped
55g/2oz anchovies, chopped (optional)
juice of 1 lemon
1 tsp ground black pepper
2 tsp olive oil

Place all the ingredients in a bowl. Mix well, or briefly blend in a blender for a smooth texture. Serve on fresh bread or as a dip with crudités.

✦OLIVE OIL AND LEMON DRINK
to soothe inflammation

2 tbsp extra virgin olive oil
juice of ½ lemon

In a cup combine the olive oil and the lemon juice. Mix well. Drink on an empty stomach every morning and wait for at least 30 minutes before having breakfast. Repeat for at least 3 weeks to notice an improvement.

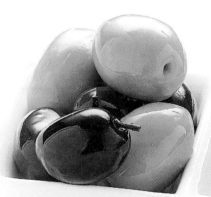

*HOT OIL TREATMENT
to treat a dry scalp and hair

125ml/4fl oz/½ cup olive oil
125ml/4fl oz/½ cup boiling water

Pour the olive oil and boiling water into a large, heatproof glass bottle or a jar with a lid. Shake well until the oil is emulsified. When the mixture has cooled slightly, massage into the hair, taking care not to burn the scalp. Put a shower cap or plastic bag over your hair and wrap it in a hot towel that has been soaked in hot water, then wrung out. Leave for about 30 minutes, then shampoo as usual.

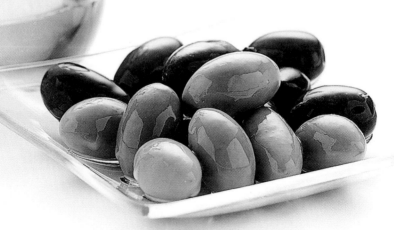

GREEK PASTA SALAD

300g/10½oz /3⅓ cups wholemeal pasta
3 tomatoes, chopped
½ cucumber, peeled and chopped
1 spring onion, trimmed and chopped
100g/3½oz/½ cup pitted black olives
55g/2oz feta cheese, cubed
5 tbsp chopped parsley
3 tbsp olive oil
salt and ground black pepper

Cook the pasta in boiling water until *al dente*, then drain. Transfer to a large bowl and add all the other ingredients. Mix well and serve.

OLIVE AND NUT DIP

225g/8oz/scant 2 cups pitted green olives
100g/3½oz/1 cup shelled walnuts
55g/2oz/⅓ cup pine nuts
2 tbsp grated Romano cheese
1 tbsp olive oil
breadsticks, to serve

Whizz the olives, walnuts and pine nuts in a blender until smooth. Mix in the grated cheese and olive oil. Serve with breadsticks.

MINI KEBABS *makes 24*

24 black olives, pitted and halved
24 cherry tomatoes, halved
48 basil leaves
24 cubes feta cheese
ground black pepper

Spear 2 olive halves, 2 tomato halves, 2 basil leaves and a cube of feta onto each of 24 cocktail sticks, alternating ingredients. Season, arrange on a serving dish and serve.

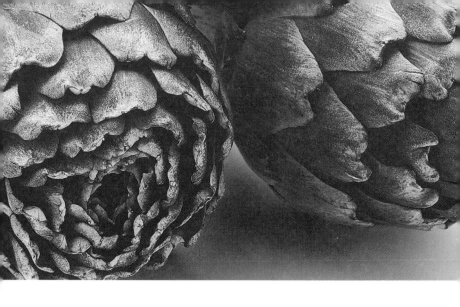

NATURE PAINTED
VEGETABLES IN A
RAINBOW OF COLOURS,
RICH IN A SPECTRUM OF
VITAMINS AND MINERALS
TO BOOST YOUR HEALTH

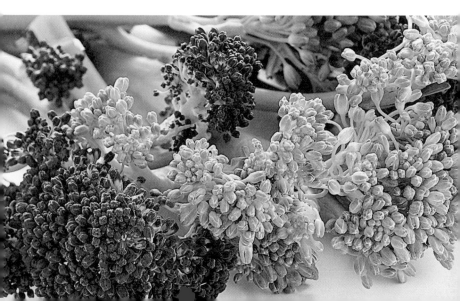

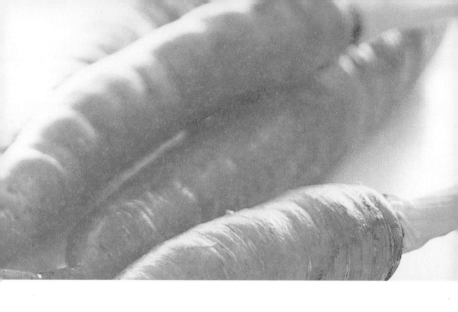

02 | wonder VEGETABLES

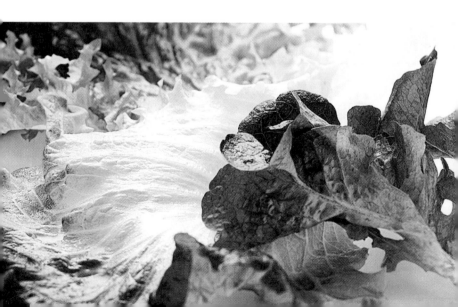

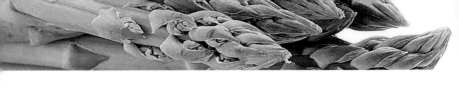

Asparagus

VITAMINS A, B1, B3, B5, C, E, K, BETA-CAROTENE, BIOTIN, FOLIC ACID; CALCIUM, COPPER, IRON, MAGNESIUM, MANGANESE, PHOSPHORUS, POTASSIUM, SELENIUM, ZINC; ASPARAGIN; GLUTATHIONE; FLAVONOIDS; FIBRE; PROTEIN

In mythology, asparagus has been renowned since ancient times both as an aphrodisiac and medicinally, for its healing properties. High in nutrients, low in calories and rich in flavour, asparagus has a wealth of health-enhancing benefits to offer.

Asparagus is a natural diuretic, encouraging the body to flush out toxins. With its active compound asparagin stimulating the kidneys, bladder and liver, asparagus is a powerful detoxifier. Its cleansing, anti-inflammatory properties make it useful for easing indigestion, irritable bowel syndrome and rheumatoid arthritis. It is also rich in the flavonoid rutin, which we need to maintain a healthy circulation.

According to folklore, asparagus is considered to be a tonic for the reproductive system. It is a fantastic source of folic acid, which is believed to prevent damage to the arteries that supply blood to the heart and the brain. Folic acid has also demonstrated powerful anti-carcinogenic properties and is said to prevent birth defects. An average portion of asparagus provides two-thirds of the daily amount of folic acid recommended for most people.

Asparagus is a rich source of beta-carotene, vitamin C and the anti-oxidant glutathione, which all lower the risk of heart disease and cancer. The vegetable is also high in antioxidant vitamin E, which fights wrinkles and premature aging, protects the heart and keeps the brain young.

Eating asparagus is said to give a natural high. The spears not only taste delicious but also supply numerous minerals and vitamins, including many of the B-vitamins, which play a central role in supporting brain function and the nervous system. If any of these are in short supply, you may be tired, depressed, anxious or constantly on edge. This can happen quite easily if you're not eating a wide range of healthy foods. B-vitamins work best together, rather than individually, keeping energy levels high and supporting mental and emotional health.

ASPARAGUS WITH HONEY AND GARLIC

450g/1lb asparagus spears, trimmed
1 tsp mustard
2 tbsp clear honey
2 garlic cloves, crushed
½ tsp chopped thyme

Steam the asparagus for 5 minutes until just tender. Drain and put on a plate. Mix together the mustard, honey, garlic and thyme, and pour over the asparagus. Serve immediately.

BALSAMIC ROASTED ASPARAGUS

500g/1lb 2oz large asparagus spears, trimmed
2 tbsp extra virgin olive oil
salt and freshly ground pepper
2 tbsp balsamic vinegar
grated lemon zest, to garnish

Preheat the oven to 400°F/200°C/gas mark 6. Coat the asparagus spears in the olive oil and season with salt and pepper. Roast on foil on a baking tray for 20–25 minutes, turning them 2–3 times. Drizzle with balsamic vinegar. Garnish with lemon zest.

✦ ASPARAGUS TINCTURE
for inflammatory conditions

10 young asparagus spears, trimmed
500ml /17fl oz/2 cups vodka

Chop the asparagus and place in a glass jar. Cover in vodka and seal the jar tightly. Stand in a dark, cool place for 10 days, then discard the asparagus. Take 8–10 drops with 1 tablespoon of water three times a day, as needed.

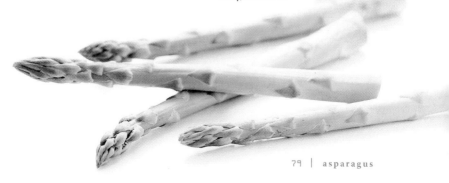

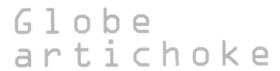

Globe artichoke

VITAMINS B1, B2, B3, B5, B6, C, E, K, BETA-CAROTENE, BIOTIN, FOLIC ACID; CALCIUM, COPPER, IRON, MAGNESIUM, MANGANESE, PHOSPHORUS, POTASSIUM, SELENIUM, ZINC; CYNARIN; FLAVONOIDS; FIBRE

This attractive and sophisticated vegetable is a form of thistle and a member of the daisy family. Recognized mostly for its detoxifying effects, globe artichoke protects the liver and supports the gallbladder, making it a useful vegetable for many traditional remedies.

Originating in the Mediterranean, artichokes are the unopened flower buds of a perennial plant. Each bud consists of several parts: outer leaves that are tough and inedible at the tip but fleshy and tender at the base; an inedible choke, or thistle, which is enclosed within a light-coloured cone of immature leaves; and a round, firm-fleshed base, known as the heart. Both the leaves and heart have a long history of therapeutic use.

Globe artichokes have traditionally been used as a hangover remedy and have detoxifying qualities. They are also valuable as a diuretic, helping to relieve water retention and high blood pressure. This makes them a useful addition to the diet of people suffering from conditions such as gout, arthritis and rheumatism. They have been used to lower blood sugar and to help to lower high cholesterol levels by inhibiting the production of more cholesterol. The antioxidant flavonoids they contain also help to keep the arteries healthy.

The ancient Greeks and Romans saw globe artichokes as a valuable digestive aid, and modern research has shown that their compound cynarin encourages the breakdown of fat as well as increasing the flow of bile and improving liver function. The hearts are particularly good for combating indigestion if eaten at the beginning of a meal. Cynarin also reduces the risk of gallstones and eases irritable bowel syndrome.

The high levels of B-vitamins in artichokes are beneficial for boosting energy and mental alertness, and together with their vitamin C, play an important role in strengthening the immune system.

ARTICHOKE SALAD

8 artichokes
4 large tomatoes, cut into wedges
1 red onion, finely sliced
½ green pepper, deseeded and chopped
100g/3½oz/½ cup green olives
1 garlic clove, crushed
6 tbsp olive oil
4 tbsp lemon juice
1 tsp Dijon mustard
salt and ground black pepper

If using fresh artichokes, break off the outer leaves and cut away the inner leaves. Scrape out the chokes and boil the hearts for about 20 minutes until tender. Rinse under cold water and combine in a large bowl with the tomatoes, onion, green pepper and olives. Whisk the remaining ingredients to make the dressing, drizzle over the vegetables and serve.

HOT ARTICHOKE DIP WITH PITTA BREAD

8 pitta breads
225g/8oz cream cheese
350g/12oz mozzarella cheese
200g/7oz/1 cup mayonnaise
150g/5½oz/1 cup grated Parmesan cheese
1 onion, finely chopped
2 garlic cloves, crushed
375g/13oz/2½ cups marinated
  artichoke hearts

Preheat the oven to 180˚C/350˚F/gas mark 4. Cut the pitta breads into small triangles, and bake on a tray for about 10 minutes. Combine the other ingredients in a food processor and whizz. Put the mixture in a dish, and cook in the oven for 30 minutes. Serve hot with the pitta dippers.

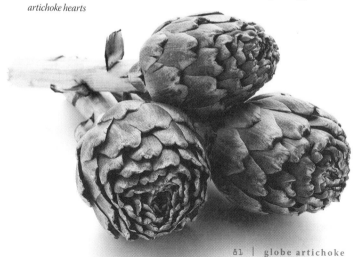

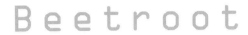

Beetroot

VITAMINS B3, B5, C, FOLIC ACID, BETA-CAROTENE; CALCIUM, COPPER, IODINE, IRON, MAGNESIUM, MANGANESE, PHOSPHORUS, POTASSIUM, SILICA, ZINC; BETANIN; FIBRE; CARBOHYDRATE

A powerful detoxifier and blood purifier, the root vegetable beetroot is rich in many nutrients crucial for immunity. It's deliciously sweet yet low in calories, and its high natural sugar content is excellent for reviving flagging energy levels.

A descendant of the sea beet that grows around the Mediterranean coast, beetroot has long been prized for its medicinal qualities, particularly for purifying the blood. It is thought that beetroot was first used in Roman times but initially utilised as a cooking ingredient by French chefs in the eighteenth century, when they introduced it in dishes. Today, there are many great ways to include this vegetable in the diet, including grating it raw into salads and adding chunks to slow-cooking soups and stews.

The brilliant ruby hue of beetroot has given it a traditional reputation as a blood purifier and great cleanser, especially of the liver, intestines, kidneys and gall bladder. It certainly aids cell cleansing by increasing the liver's production of detoxifying enzymes, and the betacyanin that makes beetroot red has antiviral and antioxidant properties and is particularly effective in combating cancerous changes, too.

The high amount of fibre contained in beetroot improves digestive health, aiding the absorption of food and helping to regulate bodily processes – two key factors in successful weight loss. It also stimulates the circulatory system, speeding up metabolism.

A rich source of natural sugars, beetroot provides easily digestible carbohydrates. Its dietary fibre slows down the absorption of these carbohydrates into the blood, which means the body is supplied with a steady stream of energy. Betacyanin also boosts the activity of natural antioxidant enzymes in the body, which protect cells against the dangers of free radical damage.

Beetroot is high in assimilable iron, and may help conditions such as anaemia, heart problems, constipation and liver toxicity, as well as restlessness and anxiety. The iron in beetroot enhances the production of disease-fighting antibodies, white blood cells (including phagocytes). It also stimulates red blood cells and improves the supply of oxygen to cells. Beetroot also contains manganese, which is needed for the formation of interferon, a powerful anti-cancer substance. In addition, it contains silica, which is vital for healthy skin, hair, fingernails, ligaments, tendons and bones.

As effective cooked as it is raw, fresh beetroot can be juiced, used in salads or made into soup. Beetroot is a popular component of juice fasts, when mixed with a sweeter juice such as apple to dilute the taste. Scientists have found that the juice combats the effects of nitrates – chemical preservatives in processed meats that can cause colon cancer. This nutrient-rich vegetable also makes an excellent detox juice, especially when mixed with carrot, spinach and cabbage.

GINGERED BEETROOT

4 beetroot (with tops), scrubbed and chopped
2 tsp sesame seeds
1 tbsp light soy sauce
1 tbsp extra virgin olive oil
1 tbsp finely chopped root ginger
100g/3½oz/¾ cup grated carrots

Steam the beetroot over a high heat for 30–40 minutes until tender. Steam the tops for 3–4 minutes, until wilted. Toast the sesame seeds in a dry pan until browned. Then, in a bowl, whisk together the soy sauce, olive oil and ginger, add all the other ingredients and toss well. Serve warm, or as a salad dish.

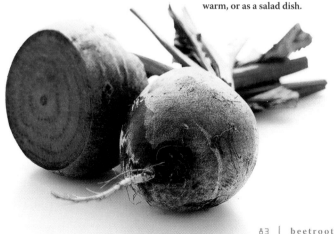

RAINBOW ROOT SALAD

2 large cooked beetroot, peeled and grated

3 carrots, peeled and grated

1 parsnip, peeled and grated

1 red onion, grated

juice of 1 lemon

1 tbsp olive oil

Mix the grated vegetables well in a large bowl. Drizzle over the lemon juice and oil, then serve.

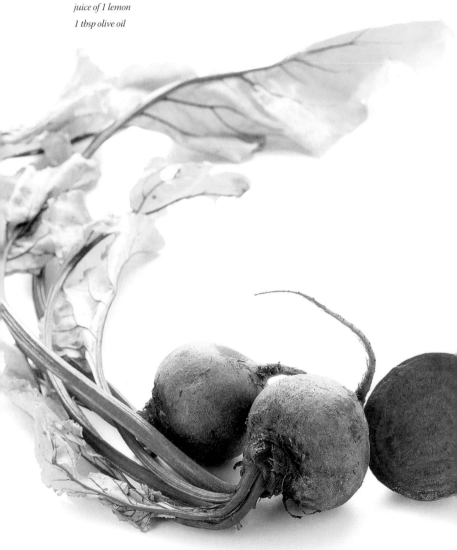

ROASTED BEETROOT

4 beetroot, washed (unpeeled)
1 tbsp olive oil
1 tsp salt

Preheat the oven to 180°C/350°F/gas mark 4. Brush the beetroot with a little olive oil, sprinkle with salt and roast for about 1 hour (depending on size). When cooked, a skewer or knife tip will easily slice into the flesh. The roasted beetroot will serve 4 as an accompaniment or 2 when sliced over a green salad.

BEETROOT SOUP

2 tbsp olive oil
1 onion, chopped
2 garlic cloves, crushed
4 large beetroot, peeled and chopped
2 carrots, peeled and chopped
1l/35fl oz/4 cups stock
4 tbsp plain bio-yogurt

Heat the oil in a large pan and fry the onion for 2–3 minutes, then add the garlic and cook for another minute. Add the beetroot, carrots and stock and bring to the boil. Cover and simmer gently for about 45 minutes, until cooked. Purée, then divide into bowls and top with the yogurt.

RAW BEETROOT SALAD

2 beetroot
½ celeriac
1 carrot
2 tbsp sunflower seeds
1 tbsp chopped parsley
2 tbsp chopped chives
4 tbsp plain bio-yogurt
1 tbsp olive oil
1 tbsp lemon juice
salt and ground black pepper

Peel and grate the beetroot, celeriac and carrot and put them in a large bowl with the sunflower seeds and herbs. Mix together using your hands, then add the remaining ingredients and mix well.

Carrot

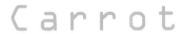

VITAMINS: B1, B3, B5, B6, C, E, K, ALPHA-CAROTENE, BETA-CAROTENE, BIOTIN, FOLIC ACID, LYCOPENE; CALCIUM, CHROMIUM, IODINE, IRON, MAGNESIUM, MANGANESE, PHOSPHORUS, POTASSIUM, SELENIUM, SILICA, ZINC; BIOFLAVONOIDS; LIMONIN; FIBRE

Carrots are packed with nutrients, which are particularly beneficial for eye health and vision. Known for their ability to aid night vision, these versatile root vegetables can be used in both sweet and savoury dishes or pressed into a delicious, sweet juice.

Arriving in Britain as early as the sixteenth century, carrots have become well known for their cleansing effect on the blood and liver, and for their ability to boost eyesight.

Carrots are among the richest sources of beta-carotene, which is converted by the body into the antioxidant vitamin A to help to prevent heart disease and speed up post-exercise recovery time. Besides giving carrots their reputation for aiding vision, beta-carotene promotes healthy digestion and protects against cancer. It's also of great benefit to the skin, and helps to strengthen cells against viruses and infections such as colds and bronchitis. Carrots are also full of the antioxidant vitamins C and E, which are crucial for supporting immunity and fighting the damaging and aging effects of free radicals.

Carrots contain vitamin K, which we use for bloodclotting and the healing of wounds, while their fibre content aids digestion and keeps the heart healthy. The chromium found in carrots helps to stabilize bloodsugar levels, making them useful for controlling diabetes and sugar cravings, and the highly concentrated sugars in carrots are easily absorbed for on-the-spot energy. The silica content of carrots is valuable for keeping the skin youthful. The vegetables are also loaded with fibre and water, which cleanse the liver, boost detoxification and plump out the skin to stave off wrinkles. They are also recommended for increasing red blood cells and are said to be useful in treating jaundice and eczema.

Carrots are fibrous root vegetables, which have tough cell walls that do not give up their nutrients easily, so to get the full nutritional value

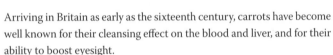

from them, carrots should be juiced or cooked rather than eaten raw. Try grating them into cakes, chopping them into stews, soups and stir-fries – cooking them in oil allows the body to use more beta-carotene. However, nibbling on raw carrot sticks and drinking the juice also have benefits, as eating just two raw carrots a day appears to reduce high cholesterol levels. This is likely to be due to calcium pectate, a type of soluble fibre that provides them with their characteristic crunchiness.

CARROT CAKE

115g/4oz butter, plus extra for greasing
115g/4oz/½ cup clear honey
115g/4oz/½ cup brown sugar
225g/8oz/1⅔ cups wholemeal flour
1 tsp baking powder
225g/8oz carrots, peeled and grated
1 tsp ground cinnamon

Grease a 20cm/8in round cake tin. In a bowl, beat the butter, honey and sugar. Fold in the remaining ingredients and spoon into the tin. Bake in a pre-heated oven at 180°C/350°F/gas mark 4 for 1 hour until firm. Remove from the oven, leave to cool, then turn out onto a wire rack.

CARROTS IN ORANGE

450g/1lb carrots, cut into batons
1 tbsp olive oil
200g/7oz onions, chopped
1 tsp caraway seeds
4 tbsp orange juice

Parboil the carrots for 5 minutes, then drain. Heat the oil in a pan and sauté the onion for 3 minutes, then add the caraway seeds for 2 minutes. Add the carrots, pour the juice over and turn up the heat until the juice boils. Reduce the heat and simmer for 5 minutes, until most of the fluid has evaporated. Serve immediately.

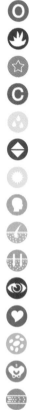

Potato

VITAMINS B1, B3, B5, B6, C, K, BIOTIN, FOLIC ACID; CALCIUM, COPPER, IODINE, IRON, MAGNESIUM, MANGANESE, PHOSPHORUS, POTASSIUM, SELENIUM, ZINC; CHLOROGENIC ACID; FIBRE; PROTEIN, CARBOHYDRATE

Simple yet immensely versatile, the potato is the world's number one vegetable crop and has long been used as a folk remedy. This staple food is packed with vitamins and many other health-giving nutrients.

Potatoes are one of the cheapest and most readily available sources of vitamin C – a nutrient that is vital for keeping the immune system healthy by fighting off damaging free radicals. It also fends off viruses that cause common ailments, such as colds, coughs and flu. New potatoes are richer in this important antioxidant than old ones. Most of the fibre, which aids digestion and lowers cholesterol, is found in the skin. Their potassium content means they can help to control high blood pressure.

Don't overlook the value of potatoes if you're aiming to get fit. They're rich in vitamin B6, which – among many other essential services – is needed to mobilize the body's glycogen stores. Vitamin B6 is also needed by phagocytes to mop up waste matter from cells and to make the immunity-boosting amino acids that are crucial for good health.

Potatoes are packed with complex carbohydrates, the best form of energy food. Complex carbs play two roles, both essential to fitness. By providing slow-burning fuel, they give you enough energy to complete your workout or match without flagging halfway through. And they help the body to maintain the muscle it has built.

Potato peel also contains a substance called chlorogenic acid, which is an anti-carcinogenic compound. In fact, peeling removes many nutrients, so try to eat potatoes in their skins.

GARLIC MASH

6 potatoes, peeled and diced

5 garlic cloves

300ml/10½fl oz/ scant 1¼ cups milk
  or soya milk

4 tbsp olive oil

1 tsp salt

a pinch of ground black pepper

1 tsp ground nutmeg

In a heavy-based pan, boil the potatoes and garlic in the milk until tender, topping up with enough water to cover them. Drain well. Add the olive oil, salt, pepper and nutmeg, then mash until smooth. Serve as a side dish.

✦ POTATO JUICE *for healthy digestion*

250g/9oz potatoes

lemon juice, to taste

Scrub and peel the potatoes, then chop into bite-sized pieces before whizzing in a blender to a fine purée. Add lemon juice to taste. Take 2 tablespoons before each meal. Do not take for longer than 24 hours.

TUNISIAN POTATOES WITH EGGS

4 eggs

450g/1lb potatoes, diced

juice of 1 lemon

2 tbsp ground cumin

2 tbsp olive oil

½ tsp harissa

Boil the eggs for 10 minutes. Leave to cool, then peel and chop. Meanwhile, boil the potatoes for 5–10 minutes until tender, then drain. Mix together the remaining ingredients and pour over the potatoes. Place on top of the eggs and serve immediately.

Sweet potato

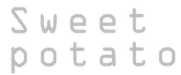

VITAMINS B1, B3, B5, B6, C, E, BETA-CAROTENE, BIOTIN, FOLIC ACID; CALCIUM, COPPER, IODINE, IRON, MAGNESIUM, MANGANESE, PHOSPHORUS, POTASSIUM, SELENIUM, ZINC; FIBRE; PROTEIN; CARBOHYDRATE

Discovered by Columbus in the West Indies, orange-fleshed sweet potatoes are packed full of beta-carotene and other nutrients. From soups, casseroles and salads to baby food and desserts, sweet potatoes add taste, valuable nutrients and colour to any meal.

Sweet potatoes are extremely rich in antioxidants. They are rich in both beta-carotene (a carotenoid with anti-viral, anti-cancer and antioxidant properties), which the body converts to vitamin A, and vitamin C, which boosts immunity and helps to prevent cardiovascular disease. These two powerful antioxidants also stave off some age-related conditions, particularly those of the eyes. Sweet potatoes are one of the few foods containing both vitamins C and E, which work synergistically with one another to help to stave off wrinkles, and to protect the eyes and preserve the memory.

Beta-carotene plays an important role in vision, bone growth, reproduction and keeping the lining of the digestive and respiratory tracts healthy, and can reduce the risk of cancer, especially endometrial cancer. For those with respiratory problems, antioxidant vitamin C acts on the lining of the lungs and makes breathing easier. Vitamin E is vital for healthy skin.

Full of fibre, especially the skin, this vegetable can help to lower cholesterol and enhance digestive function. Sweet potatoes are a complex carbohydrate and despite the name "sweet", they contain blood-sugar-regulating properties, which makes them a useful food for diabetics.

So how can something that provides all the comfort of sweetness and carbohydrates be good for you? This cheery tuber is packed with folic acid, which helps to raise your spirits. It is rich in iron and vitamin B6, so can offset any deficiency, especially for women during their periods. This vital vitamin alleviates premenstrual syndrome and food cravings, as well as helping to relieve depression. It also helps to prevent mood swings, boost the memory and protect the heart.

Sweet potatoes are low in fat and loaded with potassium, which helps to maintain fluid balance in cells, making them a useful food for dieters. An oven-baked sweet potato is the perfect light meal for anyone heading off to the gym for a workout. Always buy orange sweet potatoes – the ones with red skins – as the white variety contain far less beta-carotene.

SWEET POTATO MASH

4 sweet potatoes, peeled and chopped
3 carrots, peeled and chopped
150g/5½oz/1 cup frozen peas
30g/1oz butter
salt and ground black pepper

Steam the sweet potatoes, carrots and peas for 20–25 minutes until soft. Transfer to a bowl, add the butter and salt and pepper, and mash until creamy. Serve instead of mashed regular potatoes.

SWEET POTATO SUMMER SALAD

3 sweet potatoes baked in their skins,
*   peeled and diced*
4 spring onions, trimmed and sliced
2 celery sticks, trimmed and sliced
70g/2½oz/½ cup walnuts, chopped
1 green pepper, deseeded and sliced
200ml/7fl oz crème fraiche
2 tbsp white wine vinegar

Place all the ingredients in a large salad bowl and mix together thoroughly. Serve as a side dish.

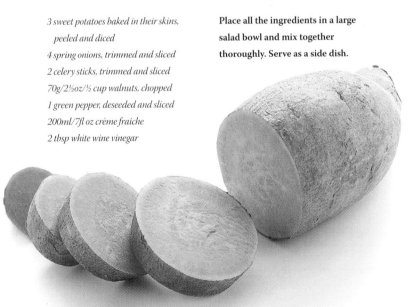

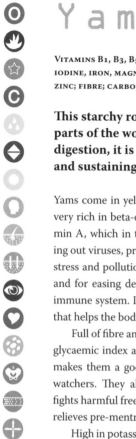

Yam

VITAMINS B1, B3, B5, B6, C, E, BETA-CAROTENE, BIOTIN, FOLIC ACID; CALCIUM, IODINE, IRON, MAGNESIUM, MANGANESE, PHOSPHORUS, POTASSIUM, SELENIUM, ZINC; FIBRE; CARBOHYDRATE

This starchy root vegetable has been a staple food in many parts of the world for centuries. Packed with fibre to aid digestion, it is an excellent power food and a delicious and sustaining form of slow-releasing carbohydrate.

Yams come in yellow, white and purple varieties, the yellow one being very rich in beta-carotene. This is needed by the body to produce vitamin A, which in turn is vital for strengthening cell membranes, keeping out viruses, preventing cancer and assisting the body in dealing with stress and pollution. Its vitamin B1 is useful for boosting energy levels, and for easing depression and stress, both of which can suppress the immune system. It is also a good source of manganese, a trace mineral that helps the body with the metabolism of carbohydrates.

Full of fibre and used in a similar way to potatoes, yams have a lower glycaemic index and so provide a more sustained form of energy. This makes them a good source of carbohydrate for diabetics and weight-watchers. They also contain vitamin C, a powerful antioxidant that fights harmful free radicals and boosts immunity, and vitamin B6, which relieves pre-mentrual symptoms.

High in potassium and low in sodium, yams help to regulate the fluid balance that exercise can so easily deplete through perspiration. Discoretine, a chemical found in yams, is particularly useful for athletes, as it reduces blood sugar and increases blood flow through the kidneys. This promotes the excretion of excess salt, which in turn helps to reduce high blood pressure.

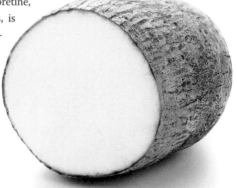

YAM AND SPINACH MASH

500g/1lb 2oz yams, peeled and diced
250g/9oz spinach
3 tbsp olive oil
1 onion, sliced
salt and ground black pepper

In a saucepan, boil the yam for 20 minutes until tender, then mash and set aside. In another pan, place the spinach in hot water and allow to wilt. Heat the oil in a frying pan and fry the onion until soft. Add the yam and spinach, combining them well. Season and serve as a side dish.

CITRUS YAMS

2 yams, peeled and chopped into
  2.5cm/1in chunks
4 tbsp olive oil
1 tbsp chopped parsley
1 tbsp chopped coriander
juice and grated zest of 1 orange
juice and grated zest of 1 lime

In a steamer or a saucepan, steam the yam for 20 minutes until tender. In a bowl, whisk together the oil, parsley and coriander, and the juice and zest of the orange and lime. Fold the cooked yam into the dressing. Serve as a starter, a side-dish or a snack.

YAM DUMPLINGS ROLLED IN POPPY SEEDS

1 yam, peeled and chopped into 2.5cm/1in
  chunks
3 egg yolks
½ tsp chilli powder
1 tsp cornflour
3 tbsp self-raising flour
4 tbsp poppy seeds

In a pan, boil the yam for 20 minutes until tender. Drain, allow to cool, then purée in a food processor. Transfer to a bowl and mix in the egg yolks, chilli powder, cornflour and flour. Form into balls and roll in the poppy seeds. Line a steamer with foil and place over a pan of simmering water. Add the dumplings and steam for 10 minutes, then serve.

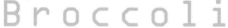

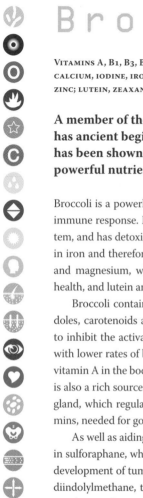

Broccoli

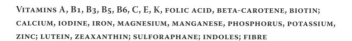

VITAMINS A, B1, B3, B5, B6, C, E, K, FOLIC ACID, BETA-CAROTENE, BIOTIN; CALCIUM, IODINE, IRON, MAGNESIUM, MANGANESE, PHOSPHORUS, POTASSIUM, ZINC; LUTEIN, ZEAXANTHIN; SULFORAPHANE; INDOLES; FIBRE

A member of the cabbage family (Cruciferae), broccoli has ancient beginnings, dating back to Roman times. It has been shown to aid many conditions, packing a more powerful nutrient punch than any other vegetable.

Broccoli is a powerhouse of antioxidant vitamin C, which is crucial for immune response. It's also full of fibre, vital for a healthy digestive system, and has detoxifying properties to help to cleanse the liver. It is rich in iron and therefore helps to treat anaemia. Broccoli contains calcium and magnesium, which stave off osteoporosis and are vital for bone health, and lutein and zeaxanthin, which reduce the risk of eye disease.

Broccoli contains a number of chemical compounds, including indoles, carotenoids and the vitamin A precursor, beta-carotene, known to inhibit the activation of cancer cells and which has been associated with lower rates of both heart and eye disease. As broccoli can increase vitamin A in the body, it also helps to improve various skin conditions. It is also a rich source of carotenoids, which are important for the thymus gland, which regulates the immune system, and is packed with B-vitamins, needed for good immune and nervous system health.

As well as aiding the body's detoxification processes, broccoli is rich in sulforaphane, which strengthens cells to resist damage and fights the development of tumours. Sulforaphane works with another compound, diindolylmethane, to inhibit cancer growth and promote antiviral and anti-bacterial activity. It has been found to improve digestion by fighting the tough bacterium *Helicobacter pylori*, which eats away at the stomach lining and can create ulcers. Broccoli counteracts these painful effects, and may even reduce the amount of harmful bacteria in the stomach.

Packed with nutrients, broccoli is also a brilliant energy-reviver. Its zinc enhances mental alertness, vitamin B5 helps the body to metabolize fats into energy and the folic acid encourages the production of serotonin, a mood-lifting chemical in the brain.

BROCCOLI STIR-FRY *serves 2*

2 tbsp sesame oil

5cm/2in piece root ginger, peeled and
  grated

1 broccoli head, chopped

1 garlic clove, crushed

Heat the oil in a frying pan, then add the ginger and broccoli. Stir-fry for 3 minutes, before adding the garlic. Contine to cook for another 2 minutes. Serve immediately, as a side dish.

WARM BROCCOLI AND SESAME SALAD

1 broccoli head, separated into florets

2 tbsp olive oil

4 tbsp soy sauce

4 tbsp rice wine vinegar

2 tbsp sesame oil

4 tbsp toasted sesame seeds

Preheat the oven to 200˚C/ 375˚F/ gas mark 5. Blanch the broccoli for 1 minute. Drain, spread on a baking tray and coat with olive oil. Roast for 10 minutes. Transfer to a bowl. Whisk the soy sauce, vinegar and sesame oil. Stir in 3 tablespoons sesame seeds. Pour over the broccoli. Sprinkle with the remaining seeds.

CHINESE-STYLE BROCCOLI

600g/1lb 5oz broccoli

100g/3½oz/½ cup tinned, sliced
  water chestnuts

2 tbsp sunflower oil

1cm/½in root ginger, peeled
  and grated

a pinch of grated lemon zest

1 tsp soy sauce

125ml/4½fl oz/
  ½ cup water

½ chicken stock
  cube

Cut the broccoli into florets. Put the water chestnuts, oil, ginger and lemon zest in a saucepan. Heat, add the broccoli and toss for 1 minute. Add the rest of the ingredients. Bring to the boil, then cover and simmer for 5 minutes. Serve immediately.

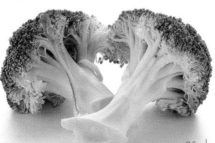

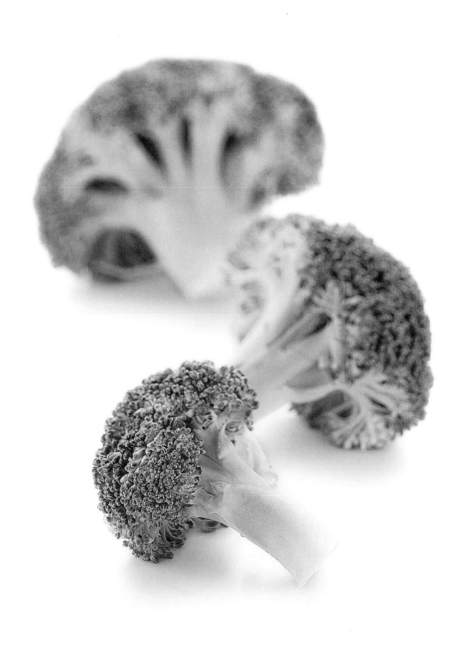

BROCCOLI WITH ALMONDS

450g/1lb broccoli florets
1 tsp olive oil
55g/2oz/⅔ cup flaked almonds
juice of 1 lemon
2 tbsp broccoli sprouts (optional)

Steam the broccoli florets for 5–10 minutes until they are just tender. Meanwhile, heat the olive oil in a pan over a low heat and fry the flaked almonds until brown. Mix together the broccoli and almonds in a serving dish and sprinkle with the lemon juice. Top the dish with broccoli sprouts, if using.

BROCCOLI POTAGE

1 tbsp olive oil
2 shallots, peeled and finely chopped
1 garlic clove, crushed
1 sweet potato, peeled and diced
1 tomato, chopped
750ml/26fl oz/3 cups vegetable stock
100g/3½oz broccoli, chopped
croutons, to serve

Heat the oil in a pan and gently fry the shallots, garlic, sweet potato and tomato for 2–3 minutes or until browned. Add the stock and broccoli, bring to the boil, then reduce the heat and simmer, covered, for 20 minutes. Pour the mixture into a blender and whizz until smooth. Return to the pan and heat through. Serve with croutons.

SPICY BROCCOLI

2 broccoli heads, broken into florets
1 onion, finely chopped
2 tbsp sunflower oil
1 tbsp curry powder
½ tsp chilli powder
250ml/9fl oz/1 cup single cream
55g/2oz/⅔ cup flaked almonds

Steam the broccoli for 6–8 minutes until tender. In another pan, fry the onion in the oil until soft. Add the broccoli, spices and cream, and simmer for 5 minutes. Scatter with the almonds. Serve as a side dish.

Kale

Vitamins B2, B3, B6, B12, C, E, K, beta-carotene, folic acid, lutein; calcium, copper, iron, magnesium, manganese, potassium, silica, zinc;
flavonoids, glucosinolates, fibre;

This leafy winter superfood will help to keep you healthy through the coldest time of the year. Bursting with vitamins and phytochemicals, kale is one of the top vegetable immunity-boosters.

Curly kale is thought to have originated in the Mediterranean region. Like cabbage and Brussels sprouts, it is a member of the Cruciferous family, sharing with these vegetables the ability to retain high levels of water and nutrients in its leaves, which makes it a very beneficial food. Curly kale can be eaten raw, steamed and served as a side dish, or lightly stir-fried. As it is in season in winter, it makes a nutritious addition to the diet during the colder months.

Kale is rich in everything from carotenoids and B-vitamins to a host of anti-aging and beautifying trace minerals. It is exceptionally high in beta-carotene, which the body turns into vitamin A. If you're a smoker, or a passive smoker, kale can help to protect your lungs from damage. A compound in cigarette smoke has been found to cause vitamin A deficiency, which can lead to lung diseases including emphysema and cancer. But foods rich in beta-carotene can counteract these effects. Kale is also one of the best sources of lutein and zeaxanthin, carotenoids that help to prevent eye disease. And the vitamins B6 and B12 in kale help to boost brain power and prevent memory loss, improve energy and bolster the immune system's ability to mop up invader cells.

A valuable source of calcium for the bones, kale also contains silica for the skin, hair, teeth and nails. Kale has high levels of glucosinolates – natural plant chemicals that block cancer-causing substances, stimulate detoxifying and repair enzymes in the body and suppress cancer cell division. It also contains flavonoids, needed for healthy circulation and to stimulate immune response, and plant sterols, important for keeping cholesterol levels low. It has high levels of antioxidant vitamin C, making it a potent defender against colds and viruses. Its anti-inflammatory effects also reduce the risk of asthma attacks and joint pains. It contains vitamin K, which promotes blood clotting and healing, and good amounts of immunity-boosting minerals, including iron and zinc.

Kale is a good source of fibre, which aids digestion and keeps blood-sugar levels steady. And all this comes for less than 45 calories a portion. Meanwhile, its long-term benefits as an antioxidant, cleansing free radicals and reducing the risk of cancer, are stacked up in your favour, too.

SESAME KALE

1 tbsp sesame oil
2 garlic cloves, crushed
450g/1lb kale, roughly chopped
1 tsp soy sauce
1 tbsp toasted sesame seeds

Heat the oil in a pan and sauté the garlic for 30 seconds over a moderate heat. Add the kale leaves and 2 tablespoons of water and increase the heat, stirring frequently until the water has evaporated. Stir in the soy sauce and the sesame seeds just before serving.

KALE WITH GARLIC AND RED PEPPERCORNS

450g/1lb kale, chopped
2 tbsp extra virgin olive oil
½ small onion, finely chopped
2 garlic cloves, crushed
½ tsp salt
½ tsp ground black pepper
¼ tsp crushed red peppercorns

Put the kale in a saucepan and cover with boiling water. Cook for 2 minutes. Drain and press until barely moist. Put the oil in a large pan and sauté the onion and garlic over a low heat for 4–5 minutes. Stir in the kale, salt, pepper and peppercorns and cook over a medium heat for 3–4 minutes. Serve immediately.

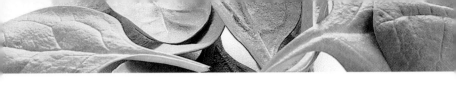

Spinach

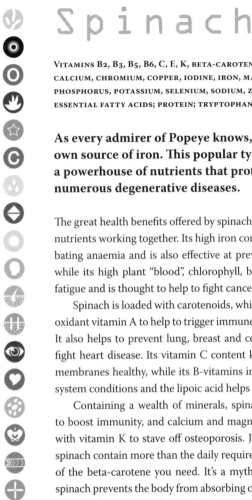

VITAMINS B2, B3, B5, B6, C, E, K, BETA-CAROTENE, BIOTIN, FOLIC ACID;
CALCIUM, CHROMIUM, COPPER, IODINE, IRON, MAGNESIUM, MANGANESE,
PHOSPHORUS, POTASSIUM, SELENIUM, SODIUM, ZINC; LIPOIC ACID; OMEGA-3
ESSENTIAL FATTY ACIDS; PROTEIN; TRYPTOPHAN; FIBRE

As every admirer of Popeye knows, spinach is nature's own source of iron. This popular type of greens contains a powerhouse of nutrients that protect the body from numerous degenerative diseases.

The great health benefits offered by spinach reside in its large number of nutrients working together. Its high iron content makes it good for combating anaemia and is also effective at preventing premature hair loss, while its high plant "blood", chlorophyll, benefits those suffering from fatigue and is thought to help to fight cancer.

Spinach is loaded with carotenoids, which the body converts to antioxidant vitamin A to help to trigger immune response to fight infections. It also helps to prevent lung, breast and cervical cancers, as well as to fight heart disease. Its vitamin C content keeps skin, hair and mucous membranes healthy, while its B-vitamins improve energy and nervous-system conditions and the lipoic acid helps to maintain the memory.

Containing a wealth of minerals, spinach is rich in zinc, required to boost immunity, and calcium and magnesium, which work together with vitamin K to stave off osteoporosis. Just 2 tablespoons of cooked spinach contain more than the daily requirement of vitamin K and most of the beta-carotene you need. It's a myth that the oxalate content of spinach prevents the body from absorbing calcium – it contains far more calcium than the oxalates can bind. Magnesium also relaxes and dilates blood vessels and helps to keep the muscles flexible.

Spinach is an anti-inflammatory and a diuretic, and can also be used to ease constipation and night blindness. Containing at least 13 flavonoid antioxidants, it may reduce the risk of heart disease and stroke. It is also rich in lutein, which guards against age-related eye diseases.

Used topically, spinach has emollient properties, helping to soften the skin and surface tissues.

SPINACH RISOTTO

1 tbsp olive oil
55g/2oz unsalted butter
2 onions, finely chopped
275g/9¾oz/1¼ cups risotto rice
1 small glass white wine
875ml/30fl oz/3½ cups vegetable stock
4 large handfuls spinach
100g/3½oz Parmesan cheese, grated

Heat the oil and butter in a pan, and lightly fry the onions until golden. Add the rice, stirring for 1 minute, then add the wine and leave until absorbed. Add enough stock to cover, leave to absorb, and keep adding until all the stock is used and the rice is cooked. Stir in the spinach and cook until wilted. Remove from heat and sprinkle with Parmesan, then serve.

✦SPINACH POULTICE *for calluses and heel spurs*

40g/1½ oz/1 cup spinach, crushed
gauze bandage

Wrap the spinach leaves in the bandage and tie to the affected area. Leave for 20 minutes, then discard. Repeat as necessary to soften and soothe inflamed or hardened tissue.

CHEESE AND SPINACH MELT

1 onion, chopped
1 tbsp olive oil
2 garlic cloves, crushed
55g/2oz/⅓ cup pine nuts
225g/8oz baby leaf spinach
250g/9oz cheese, grated

Gently fry the onion in the oil, add the garlic and pine nuts, and stir in the spinach until it wilts. Drain off any excess liquid, then add the cheese, stirring until it melts. Use the mixture in pancakes, on toast or to stuff vegetables.

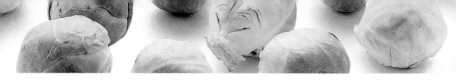

Brussels sprout

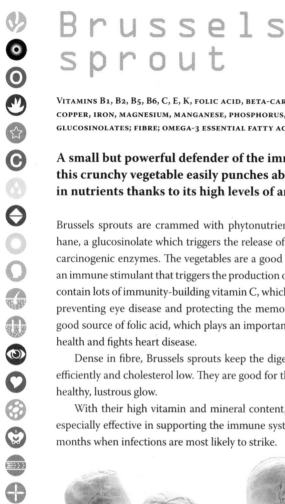

VITAMINS B1, B2, B5, B6, C, E, K, FOLIC ACID, BETA-CAROTENE; CALCIUM, COPPER, IRON, MAGNESIUM, MANGANESE, PHOSPHORUS, POTASSIUM; GLUCOSINOLATES; FIBRE; OMEGA-3 ESSENTIAL FATTY ACIDS; PROTEIN

A small but powerful defender of the immune system, this crunchy vegetable easily punches above its weight in nutrients thanks to its high levels of antioxidants.

Brussels sprouts are crammed with phytonutrients, such as sulforaphane, a glucosinolate which triggers the release of detoxifying and anticarcinogenic enzymes. The vegetables are a good source of vitamin B5, an immune stimulant that triggers the production of antibodies, and they contain lots of immunity-building vitamin C, which keeps us youthful by preventing eye disease and protecting the memory. Sprouts are also a good source of folic acid, which plays an important role in reproductive health and fights heart disease.

Dense in fibre, Brussels sprouts keep the digestive system working efficiently and cholesterol low. They are good for the skin too, giving it a healthy, lustrous glow.

With their high vitamin and mineral content, Brussels sprouts are especially effective in supporting the immune system during the winter months when infections are most likely to strike.

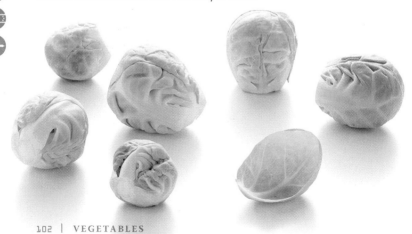

NUTTY SPROUT STIR-FRY

2 onions, sliced
150g/5½ oz/1 cup blanched almonds
4 tbsp olive oil
600g/1lb 5oz Brussels sprouts, trimmed
  and sliced
ground black pepper, to taste

Fry the onions and almonds in the oil until the onions are soft. Blanch the sprouts for 1 minute in a pan of lightly salted boiling water, then add to the pan with the onions and almonds, cooking gently until the sprouts are tender. Season to taste with black pepper and serve.

BRUSSELS SPROUTS WITH BACON

450g/1lb Brussels sprouts, trimmed
115g/4oz back bacon, diced
100g/3½oz/¼ cup roasted, salted
  pistachios, shelled
4 tbsp balsamic vinegar
salt and ground black pepper

Steam the sprouts for 5–10 minutes, until almost tender. In a frying pan, cook the bacon until crisp. Remove the bacon, add the sprouts to the pan and sauté for 1–2 minutes. Add the pistachios and vinegar, and continue to cook for 1–2 minutes, reducing the vinegar and glazing the sprouts and nuts. Return the bacon to the pan, season, mix well and serve.

BRUSSELS SPROUTS WITH CHESTNUTS

4 bacon rashers (optional)
400g/14oz Brussels sprouts, trimmed
400g/14oz chestnuts, cooked or vacuum-
  packed
25g/1oz butter
salt and ground black pepper

Grill the bacon, if using, and cut into strips. Steam or boil the sprouts for 5 minutes until cooked but still crunchy. Drain the sprouts, add the chestnuts, butter and the bacon strips, if using. Season and serve immediately.

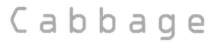

Cabbage

VITAMINS A, B1, B2, B3, B5, B6, C, E, K, U, BETA-CAROTENE, BIOTIN, FOLIC
ACID; CALCIUM, IODINE, IRON, MAGNESIUM, MANGANESE, PHOSPHORUS,
POTASSIUM, SELENIUM, SULPHUR, ZINC; FIBRE; OMEGA-3 OILS;
GLUCOSINOLATES; INDOLES, PROTEIN

**Packed with antioxidants and cancer-fighting
compounds, cabbages were used in therapeutic rituals
in ancient Greek and Roman times.**

A member of the cruciferous food family, cabbage contains powerful
anti-carcinogenic compounds, namely indoles and glucosinolates. Studies have shown that people who eat at least three servings of cruciferous
vegetables each week have a lowered risk of prostate, colorectal and lung
cancer. Indoles also help to deactivate oestrone, a dangerous form of oestrogen that is associated with breast cancer.

Cabbages are rich in antioxidant nutrients such as vitamin C, which
mops up free radicals and protects the cardiovascular system. It also
promotes healthy skin and glossy hair, and boosts immunity. Its beta-
carotene also enhances the immune system, reduces blood pressure and
fights heart disease. Cabbages provide folic acid, and may therefore help
to reduce birth defects. Their phytonutrients help the liver to remove
toxins and they also combat arthritis and eye disease. Red cabbage is
richest in vitamin C and and can help to ward off Alzheimer's disease.

A substance unique to raw cabbage known as vitamin U or S-
methylmethionine has had remarkable success in healing stomach and
duodenal ulcers within as little as
four days. And cabbage can
be a useful aid for general
gastro-intestinal health
– the German ferm-
ented cabbage dish
sauerkraut supports
the digestive tract by
promoting the growth of
friendly bacteria in the gut.

Cabbage leaves can be used placed over leg ulcers and wounds to help to heal them. Mastitis or breast inflammation, often experienced by breast-feeding mothers, may also be relieved in this way.

It is a good idea to let cruciferous vegetables stand for a few minutes after chopping them, as this creates many healthy compounds.

STIR-FRIED CABBAGE WITH FENNEL SEEDS

1 green cabbage
2 tbsp balsamic vinegar
1 tsp fennel seeds
a pinch of cayenne pepper
salt and ground black pepper

Wash the cabbage and shred it into thin strips. Put the balsamic vinegar in a wok and heat until sizzling. Add the cabbage, fennel seeds, cayenne pepper, and salt and pepper. Cook until the cabbage is softened and slightly browned.

CABBAGE AND APPLE SALAD

175g/6oz red cabbage, shredded
175g/6oz green cabbage, shredded
2 tbsp olive oil
1 tbsp lemon juice
1 garlic clove, crushed
4 apples, chopped

Mix together the shredded cabbages, olive oil, lemon juice and garlic in a large bowl. Refrigerate for at least 2 hours until ready to serve. Add the apples, season if desired and serve immediately.

✦RAW CABBAGE POULTICE
for inflammation, such as arthritis and mastitis

5 inside cabbage leaves
3 tbsp hot chamomile tea
soft cotton cloth

Chop the cabbage leaves into small pieces and place in a bowl. Add the chamomile tea and combine. Roll mixture in the cloth and apply to the inflamed area. Leave for 5 minutes. Repeat as required.

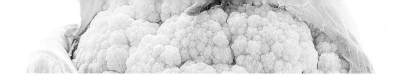

Cauliflower

VITAMINS B3, B5, B6, C, FOLIC ACID; CALCIUM, MANGANESE, POTASSIUM, ZINC;
GLUCOSINOLATES; INDOLES; OMEGA-3 ESSENTIAL FATTY ACIDS; FIBRE

Thought to have originated from China, cauliflower is a great source of health-giving phytochemicals.

Among the many health-giving attributes of cauliflower is its ability to aid cell detoxification. Processed food is full of manufactured chemicals and even healthy food can contain elements that have harmful side effects. The liver works hard to filter out these toxins, which can cause cell damage leading to cancer and other diseases, and is helped by cauliflower, which is rich in antioxidants. But cauliflower's most powerful effects come from compounds such as glucosinolates, which fuel and strengthen the liver during all stages of detoxification. The glucosinolate sulforaphane steps up the production of enzymes that sweep toxins out of the body, while Indole-3-carbinol reduces levels of harmful oestrogens that can foster tumour growth, particularly in the breast, prostate, lung, stomach and colon.

Cauliflower is high in vitamin C, folic acid and zinc, all known for boosting immunity. Vitamin C has antiviral properties, while folic acid is vital for reproductive health and zinc aids the healing of wounds. One large serving of cauliflower provides all the vitamin C you need in a day.

The most important nutrients for energy production and supporting the adrenal glands are the B-vitamins, which cauliflower has in abundance – especially B5, needed for the production of antibodies. Cauliflower also has anti-allergenic properties that can help to ease asthma and skin allergies.

INDIAN-STYLE CAULIFLOWER

1 onion, finely chopped

1 tbsp olive oil

1 garlic clove, crushed

1 tsp ground ginger

1 tsp ground coriander

1 tsp ground turmeric

1 cauliflower, cut into
   small florets

2 tbsp water

In a frying pan, gently fry the onion in the oil for 5 minutes. Add the garlic, spices, cauliflower and water. Cover and simmer, stirring occasionally, until the cauliflower is tender. Continue to cook, stirring, until the cauliflower is dry. Serve as a side dish.

CAULIFLOWER WITH PARSLEY AND RED PEPPER

1 cauliflower

60ml/2fl oz/¼ cup water

5 black olives, pitted and finely chopped

1 tbsp finely chopped parsley

1 tsp red wine vinegar

a pinch of crushed red pepper flakes

Put the cauliflower and water in a saucepan. Cover and bring to the boil. Reduce heat and cook for 4–5 minutes, or until the cauliflower starts to soften. Stir in the olives, parsley, vinegar and pepper flakes. Cook for 1 minute or until thoroughly heated through.

CAULIFLOWER PROVENÇALE

1 tbsp olive oil

1 large onion, chopped

2 garlic cloves, crushed

2 small courgettes, diced

400g/14oz tinned tomatoes

1 large cauliflower, cut
   into florets

Heat the oil and fry the onion for 2–3 minutes. Stir in the garlic, add the courgettes and tomatoes and simmer for 5–10 minutes. Meanwhile, steam the cauliflower for 5–10 minutes until tender and place in a serving dish. Pour over the sauce and serve.

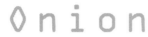

Onion

VITAMINS B1, B6, C, FOLIC ACID; CHROMIUM, COPPER, MANGANESE, MOLYBDE-
NUM, PHOSPHORUS, POTASSIUM, SELENIUM; SULPHUR COMPOUNDS; QUERCETIN,
FLAVONOIDS; FIBRE

A member of the Allium family, the onion has long played a central role in folk medicine and has a wealth of health-giving properties. As strong in healing power as it is in taste, this vegetable keeps disease at a safe distance.

The powerful anti-inflammatory effects of onions make them a vital ingredient in nourishing winter dishes. They are full of nutrients that counteract respiratory problems at all levels, from the nasal congestion caused by a cold to the wheezing of asthma. Their antibacterial action combats all kinds of infectious disease and they protect the digestive system, reducing the risk of intestinal growths that could lead to cancer. The same compounds cause the onion's smell and its healing effects, so the more pungent the onion, the more good it will do you.

Protectors of the circulatory system, onions contain many compounds that help to lower cholesterol, thin the blood and prevent the formation of clots and the hardening of arteries. They may halt the progression of cancerous tumours in the gut. Containing sulphur, an important constituent of the building blocks of skin, nails and hair, onions help to keep us looking our best. Another attribute of sulphur is that it also inhibits the body's inflammatory response, thus treating everything from insect bites to allergies.

Onions have an exceptionally high level of the flavonoid quercetin, a strong antioxidant that can block the formation of cancer cells. Quercetin is anti-inflammatory, antibiotic and antiviral and, like beta-carotene, not destroyed in cooking. These nutrient-dense vegetables are also thought to suppress the activity of the *Helicobacter pylori* bacterium, which causes stomach ulcers and food poisoning.

A good source of antioxidant Vitamin C, which fights off harmful free radicals and supports the immune system, onions are also loaded with selenium, another powerful immunity-booster, which also cleanses the liver, and staves off wrinkles and sun damage.

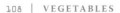

For anyone aiming to reach peak physical fitness, onions can offer several minerals, including chromium, manganese and potassium, which help to break down fat deposits and speed up the metabolism. Their quercetin has been shown to reduce muscle fatigue. Studies suggest that onions can help to maintain healthy bones by inhibiting the activity of osteoclasts – the cells that break down bone.

FRENCH ONION SOUP

4 tbsp olive oil
750g/1½lb onions, thinly sliced
2 garlic cloves, crushed
2 tbsp apple juice
1.2l/40fl oz/4¾ cups beef stock
300ml/10fl oz/1¼ cups dry white wine
salt and ground black pepper

In a heavy saucepan heat the oil. Add the onions, garlic and apple juice, and cook for 5–6 minutes, stirring constantly. Turn down the heat and cook for about 20 minutes. Pour the stock and wine into the mixture and season with salt and pepper. Bring to a simmer and cook uncovered for 1 hour. Pour into bowls and serve.

✦ONION COMPRESS
for inflamed wounds, headaches & earaches

4 onions, finely chopped
white muslin or linen bag

Lightly steam the onions and wrap in the white muslin or linen bag. Apply to the inflamed area or aching parts. Once the compress cools down, replace it with another. Repeat up to four times in succession, or until the symptoms are alleviated.

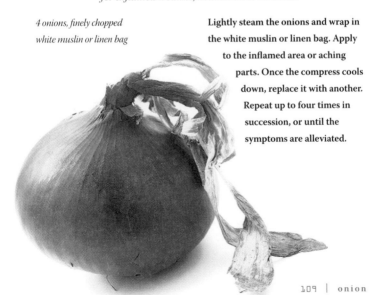

Celery

Vitamins B1, B2, B3, B5, B6, C, E, K, beta carotene, biotin, folic acid; calcium, iodine, iron, magnesium, manganese, molybdenum, phosphorus, potassium, selenium, sodium, zinc; fibre

A member of the parsley family, celery can stimulate the kidneys and help to flush out the system. Just three celery sticks make up one of the five recommended daily portions of fruit and vegetables.

Thought to have its origins in southern Europe and North Africa, celery was known as a medicine by the ancient Greeks, while its culinary uses were first explored in Europe in the Middle Ages.

Full of B-vitamins for energy and immunity-boosting Vitamin C, celery is good at aiding the elimination of waste via the urine, thus acting as a detoxifying agent, and cleansing the liver, which helps to keep skin looking youthful. It is an anti-inflammatory, clearing uric acid from painful joints, and is well known as a remedy for gout and rheumatism. Celery is a useful antiseptic in the urinary tract and may help to lower blood pressure and prevent cancer. Celery seeds are more potent than other parts of the plant.

It is believed that we burn more calories chewing, swallowing and digesting celery than we get from eating it, making the vegetable popular with dieters. Its high water content acts as a diuretic helping to eliminate puffy hands, ankles and feet.

A stick of celery is the athlete's secret weapon because it's rich in a string of nutrients that keep energy levels high. Its vitamin C content aids recovery from sports injuries by strengthening cell walls. And being higher in sodium than most vegetables (though nowhere near a harmful level), celery could prevent the dangerous mineral imbalance that results from drinking too much water during an energetic workout. Vital minerals can be lost in the sweat following vigorous exercise or during a fever. Celery juice, with its high concentration of water, potassium and naturally occurring sodium, can help to replace this loss by hydrating the body and restoring electrolyte balance. As celery juice has a strong flavour, most people prefer it mixed with other juices, such as carrot.

Celery contains a rich spectrum of other health-enhancing minerals, including calcium, iron, magnesium and selenium, which work together to normalize the body's acid–alkaline balance. An acidic state caused by stress or eating harmful foods can lead to numerous health problems. Celery seems to counteract this acidity, thereby improving conditions such as fatigue, rheumatism and joint pain.

CLASSIC WALDORF SALAD

5 celery sticks, trimmed and chopped

2 apples, chopped

1 bunch white seedless grapes

1 spring onion, trimmed and chopped

1 handful chopped walnuts

2 tbsp mayonnaise

2 tbsp plain bio-yogurt

½ tsp celery seeds

ground black pepper, to taste

Put the celery, apples, grapes, spring onion and walnuts in a large bowl. Put the remaining ingredients in a separate small bowl and stir well. Tip the mixture onto the salad and mix well. Serve immediately.

✦CELERY-SEED TEA
for rheumatism & urinary infections

1 heaped tsp celery seeds

500ml/17fl oz/2 cups water

Place the seeds and water in a stainless-steel pan. Bring to the boil, then remove from the heat and leave to infuse for 10 minutes. Strain. Drink up to 3 times a day depending on the severity of symptoms.

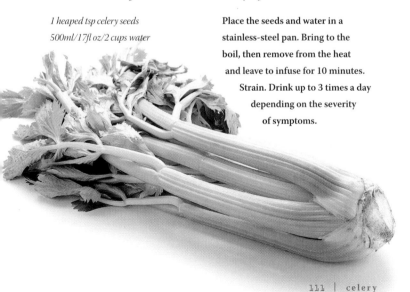

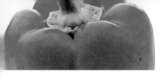
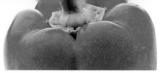
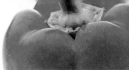

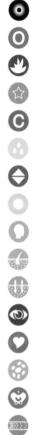

Pepper

Vitamins B3, B6, C, E, K, beta-carotene, biotin, folic acid, lycopene; calcium, iodine, iron, magnesium, manganese, phosphorus, potassium, zinc; fibre

The wide range of vitamins and minerals in this colourful vegetable makes it a great all-round immunity-booster. Whether eaten raw as a crunchy crudité or softened in a stir-fry or roasting dish, sweet peppers pack a powerful nutritional punch.

Sweet peppers come in several colours: red, green, orange, yellow and even purple. The green and purple varieties have a slightly bitter taste, while the red, yellow and orange peppers have a sweeter flavour.

Whatever their colour, they provide a healthy serving of immunity-boosting nutrients, including two antioxidants that work well together: beta-carotene and vitamin C. Together, these offer protection against cell-damaging free radicals and protect the lungs from winter infections, asthma and even the ravages of second-hand smoke. The body turns the beta-carotene into antiviral, immunity-boosting vitamin A, while vitamin C is said to protect against memory problems and eye disease, and to combat stress. Peppers also contain flavonoids, which are thought to enhance vitamin C's antioxidant action by strengthening its ability to protect the body against disease. One average serving of sweet peppers contains the daily needs of these vitamins for most people.

Red peppers are especially high in cancer-fighting lycopene, which in conjunction with the vitamin C and carotenoids, further protects vision and reduces the risk of eye diseases. Lycopene also helps to fight almost every aspect of the aging process, including deterioration of the skin structure and damage to the arteries.

With a high water content, which helps to flush out toxins from the body, sweet peppers also contain fibre, which is important for digestive health and for preventing the build up of cholesterol in the blood that can cause heart attacks and strokes. The B-vitamins in peppers also help to ward off atherosclerosis and heart disease by reducing levels of homocysteine, a substance that damages blood vessels.

STUFFED PEPPERS

3 tbsp olive oil

200g/7oz cherry tomatoes

2 garlic cloves, finely chopped

1 red onion, finely chopped

1 bunch basil, shredded

100g/3½oz mozzarella cheese, cut into
   small cubes

100g/3½oz Parmesan cheese, grated

4 red peppers, topped and deseeded

ground black pepper, to taste

Preheat the oven to 220°C/425°F/gas mark 7. Spoon 2 tablespoons of the olive oil into an ovenproof dish and place in the oven. Meanwhile, combine all the ingredients except the peppers in a bowl with the remaining olive oil. Fill each pepper with equal amounts of the mixture, then put the tops on. Place in the dish and cook for 20 minutes. Serve immediately.

ROAST PEPPER AND BASIL DIP

1 large red pepper

100ml/4fl oz/scant ½ cup milk

½ tsp paprika

½ tsp salt

2 tsp extra virgin olive oil

2 tsp cider vinegar

1 tbsp chopped basil

Preheat the oven to 200°C/400°F/gas mark 6. Put the whole pepper on a baking tray in the centre of the oven for 20–30 minutes, or until the skin goes black. Remove, and allow to cool. Peel off the skin, seed and core, and save any juice. Blend all the ingredients, including the pepper and its juice, in a food processor to a smooth creamy texture. Serve either chilled as a dip or warm as a sauce.

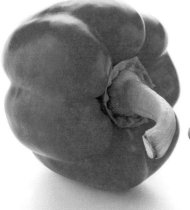

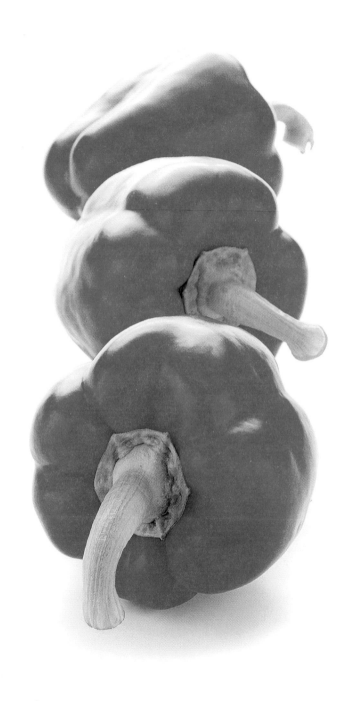

GRILLED PEPPER AND WALNUT SALAD

4 sweet peppers, deseeded and cut
   into strips
1 handful walnut halves
2 tbsp olive oil
1 tsp vinegar
1 lettuce, roughly torn
salt, to taste

Cook the peppers under a hot grill until the skin is black and blistered. When cool enough to touch, peel off the skin and discard. Heat the walnuts gently in 1 teaspoon of the oil in a frying pan until crisp. Mix together the remaining oil, vinegar and salt. Place the lettuce in a serving bowl and the peppers and walnuts on top. Pour over the dressing and serve while still warm.

RED PEPPER SAUCE

2 red peppers, deseeded and chopped
250g/9oz/1⅔ cups cashew nuts
1 tsp dried dill
1 garlic clove
1 tbsp chopped onion
pinch of ground black pepper

Put all the ingredients in a food processor and blend until creamy. Serve over rice or couscous, or steamed vegetables, or use as a sandwich spread.

RED PEPPER SALSA

1½ red peppers, deseeded and finely
   chopped
2 beef tomatoes, finely diced
1 small red pepper, deseeded and
   finely diced
1 small cucumber, finely diced
4 tbsp chopped coriander
juice and grated zest of ½ lime

Mix all the ingredients together in a bowl. Serve as a dip or a sauce.

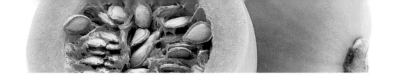

Squash

VITAMINS B1, B3, B5, B6, C, E, K, BETA CAROTENE, FOLIC ACID; CALCIUM,
COPPER, IRON, MAGNESIUM, MANGANESE, PHOSPHORUS, POTASSIUM,
SELENIUM, ZINC; FIBRE; OMEGA-3 FATTY ACIDS; PROTEIN;
COMPLEX CARBOHYDRATE

**Squash is a nutritional winner and is delicious in soups
and stews and with other roasted vegetables. A bright
orange "superveg", it gives a powerful boost to the body's
immune defences.**

The solid flesh of squash, such as butternut and pumpkin, provides a
healthy dose of age-defying nutrients. Extracts from squash have been
found to help ease the swelling of the prostate gland, which bedevils many
older men. Eating squash regularly may help to prevent it developing.
Their rich array of nutrients, including beta-cryptoxanthin, counteract
the cell damage that leads to cancer and heart disease. And they have anti-
inflammatory properties that could relieve the pain of many age-related
conditions, such as arthritis.

Like all orange fruit and vegetables, the butternut squash is a great
source of beta-carotene, which the body converts to vitamin A, needed

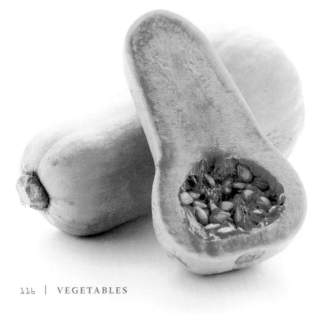

for maintaining a healthy immune system as well as for good digestion and respiratory-tract function.

A great provider of energy-sustaining carbohydrates, squash contains high levels of the minerals potassium and magnesium, which help to maintain efficient energy production. A lack of these minerals can lead to fatigue, muscle cramps and an increased risk of high cholesterol, high blood pressure and heart problems.

ROAST BUTTERNUT SQUASH WITH CHEESE AND WALNUTS

4 tbsp olive oil

2 garlic cloves, crushed

2 butternut squash, halved and deseeded

200g/7oz cheese, cubed

100g/3½ oz/1 cup walnut halves

Preheat the oven to 190°C/375°F/gas mark 5. Place the oil and garlic in the hollow of each squash. Roast the squash for 1 hour, until tender. Scoop out most of the flesh, leaving enough to keep the shape. Mix together the flesh with the cheese and walnuts. Place in the skins and cook for a few minutes until the cheese is soft. Serve immediately.

SPICY ROASTED VEGETABLES

3 tbsp sunflower seeds

1 tsp chilli powder

1 tsp cumin seeds

1 tsp ground coriander

1 tsp ground ginger

1 butternut squash, peeled and deseeded

2 courgettes, chopped

1 red pepper, deseeded and sliced

200g/7oz button mushrooms

3 tbsp olive oil

1 tbsp balsamic vinegar

Toast the sunflower seeds and spices in a frying pan over a low heat for 3 minutes. Chop the squash into 5cm/2in chunks. Place the squash and the other vegetables in an oven-proof dish. Add the oil, balsamic vinegar, seeds and spices, and mix well together. Bake in a preheated oven at 190°C/375°F/gas mark 5 for 1 hour, stirring occasionally, then serve.

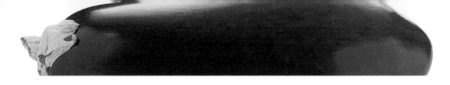

Aubergine

Vitamins B1, B3, B6, C, K, beta-carotene, biotin, folic acid; calcium, copper, iodine, iron, magnesium, manganese, phosphorus, potassium, selenium, zinc; chlorogenic acid; anthocyanins; fibre

Thanks to its high number of healing compounds, aubergine helps to ward off many illnesses. The polished purple skin of this plant has very powerful qualities.

Well-known as a main ingredient in the Greek dish moussaka, aubergines contain many beneficial substances. Some people need more iron in their diet, but too much iron isn't a good thing – it increases the body's production of free radicals, byproducts of metabolic processes that damage the cells. Aubergines contain a host of phytonutrients that mop up harmful free radicals. One of them is chlorogenic acid, a powerful antioxidant that lowers levels of harmful cholesterol and has antibacterial and antiviral properties. Another is nasunin, an anthocyanin found to protect fats in brain cells, which may help to slow down the aging process of this vital organ and which also helps the body excrete excess iron. This reduces the risk of conditions such as cancer, heart disease and arthritis.

A member of the nightshade family, aubergines should be avoided by osteoarthritis sufferers, as they may increase inflammation in the joints.

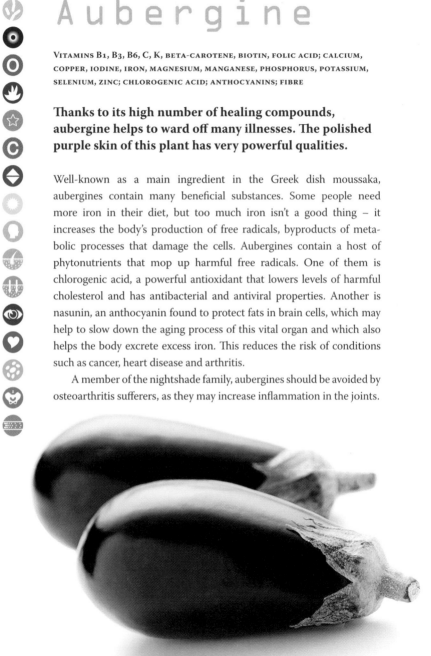

BABA GANNOUSH

2 large aubergines
6 garlic cloves, crushed
4 tbsp tahini
4 tbsp lemon juice
1 tbsp olive oil
1 bunch parsley
bread and crudités, to serve

Preheat the oven to 190°C/375°F/gas mark 5. Bake the aubergines on a baking tray for 30 minutes. Slice in half, scoop out the insides and chop. Drain in a colander for at least 10 minutes. In a bowl, mash the garlic, tahini and lemon juice with the aubergine to form a paste. Pour oil over, and sprinkle with parsley. Serve with bread and crudités.

AUBERGINE GRATIN

2 aubergines
3 tbsp olive oil
100g/3½oz Cheddar cheese or dairy-free
    alternative, grated

Preheat the oven to 220°C/425°F/gas mark 7. Cut the aubergine into slices and brush the sides with the oil. Arrange in an oven-proof dish in overlapping slices, cover with foil and cook for 25 minutes. Remove the foil and cook for a further 10 minutes. Remove from the oven, sprinkle with the cheese and place under a grill until melted.

AUBERGINE AND RICOTTA ROLLS

1 large aubergine, trimmed
3 tbsp olive oil
juice and grated zest of 1 lemon
200g/7oz ricotta cheese
4 sun-dried tomatoes, chopped
ground black pepper

Cut the aubergine lengthways into 5mm/¼in thick slices. Cover with the oil, and lemon juice and zest. Place on a baking tray and grill each side for 3 minutes. Put some ricotta, tomato and black pepper on each slice. Roll and secure with a cocktail stick. Grill for 2 minutes, then serve.

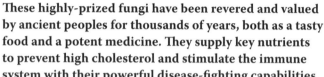

Mushroom

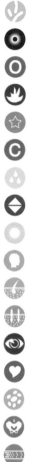

VITAMINS B1, B2, B3, B5, B6, B12, C, E, FOLIC ACID; CALCIUM, CHROMIUM, COPPER, IRON, MAGNESIUM, MANGANESE, PHOSPHOROUS, POTASSIUM, SELENIUM, ZINC; LENTINAN; L-ERGOTHIONEINE; ERITADENINE; BETA-GLUCAN; PROTEIN; OMEGA-6 ESSENTIAL FATTY ACIDS

These highly-prized fungi have been revered and valued by ancient peoples for thousands of years, both as a tasty food and a potent medicine. They supply key nutrients to prevent high cholesterol and stimulate the immune system with their powerful disease-fighting capabilities.

There are many species of mushroom available today in supermarkets. Among the more common ones are button, chestnut and Portobello mushrooms, but all species are packed with health-giving nutrients. Made up of between 80 and 90 per cent water, they are very low in calories and are therefore a useful food for dieters.

Mushrooms are one of the richest sources of a powerful antioxidant called L-ergothioneine, which combats cell damage. Research is being done into their cancer-fighting properties, including reducing the risk of breast cancer. And their minerals may ease the pain of arthritis. Mushrooms may also help to slow down age-related muscle loss, as they provide protein in a form that the body can easily use.

All mushrooms are high in B-vitamins, particularly vitamin B3, which may slow the onset of age-related dementias. They are a rich source of potassium, which helps to regulate blood pressure – one average Portobello mushroom contains more potassium than a banana. Mushrooms are also an important source of vitamin B12 for vegetarians, which is vital for maintaining healthy energy levels and combating arthritis.

Brimming with the anti-aging antioxidants vitamin E and selenium, mushrooms help to maintain healthy skin and hair, and protect against heart disease. The fungi are a slow-release energy food, thanks to their high content of vegetable protein. They're also especially rich in chromium, which helps to stabilize blood-sugar levels and, in turn, helps to control sugar cravings. The older you are, the less likely you are to be taking in enough chromium.

Shiitake mushroom: Native to China, Japan and Korea, shiitake mushrooms have been used in those countries for thousands of years to prevent and treat illness. In ancient China they were prescribed by physicians to help to beat a range of conditions, from colds and flu to gastrointestinal problems. Recently, these mushrooms have been the subject of several studies that are researching their pro-immunity and healing powers.

These fungi contain lentinan, a compound that has been shown to help lower cholesterol. Lentinan has also been isolated and licensed as an anti-cancer drug in Japan because of its ability to stimulate the immune system to deactivate malignant cells. In addition, lentinan is understood to trigger the production of the antiviral and anti-bacterial substance interferon, which may help to inhibit the progress of the HIV virus as well as treat cancer, diabetes, chronic fatigue syndrome and fibrocystic breast disease. The mushrooms are also rich in the amino acids that enhance general immune function. They contain eritadenine, a digestive enzyme which is thought to lower cholesterol, while their tyrosinase lowers blood pressure. They are also rich in iron, which staves off anaemia.

Although shiitake mushrooms are more expensive than many other varieties, a small amount gives great health benefits and satisfies the appetite. They can be bought fresh, pickled or dried, and can be used in dishes in the same way as ordinary field mushrooms.

Maitake mushroom: Another type of fungus from the Far East with excellent healing powers is the maitake mushroom. Maitake mushrooms contain beta-glucan, which stops the HIV virus from killing white blood cells, possibly preventing AIDS. Beta-glucan is known to be highly effective in shrinking cancerous tumours. Maitake mushrooms are also used to treat high blood pressure and liver disease.

Reishi mushroom: This fungus is used in extract or essence form as a treatment for liver disorders, hypertension and arthritis. Studies have shown that it has antiviral, anti-bacterial, antioxidant anti-allergic and anti-inflammatory properties, and scentists believe that it helps to fight tumours. In addition, the reishi mushroom is used to combat high blood pressure and asthma.

GLAZED SHIITAKE MUSHROOMS

450g/1lb shiitake mushrooms
1 tsp rapeseed oil
80ml/2½fl oz/⅓ cup chicken stock
1 tsp cornflour
2 tsp soy sauce
1 tbsp dry sherry

Discard the shiitake stalks and slice the mushrooms. In a large pan, heat the oil and add the mushrooms and 2 tablespoonfuls of the stock. Cook, stirring often, for 5–6 minutes. In a small bowl, dissolve the cornflour in the remaining stock. Stir in the soy sauce and sherry. Add the mixture to the pan. Cook for 2 minutes, or until the mushrooms are glazed.

MUSHROOM PÂTÉ

375g/13oz chestnut mushrooms, chopped
2 tbsp olive oil
1 tbsp soy sauce
200g/7oz mascarpone cheese
2 tbsp chopped tarragon

In a pan, fry the mushrooms in the oil for 2 minutes. Add 4 tablespoons of water and simmer for 10 minutes. Allow to cool, then drain and purée in a blender. Stir in the remaining ingredients. Refrigerate for at least 1 hour, then serve.

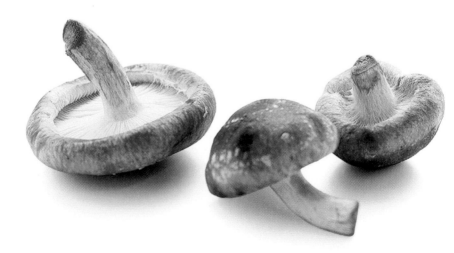

SHIITAKE NOODLES

250g/9oz thick egg noodles
3 tbsp soy sauce
1 tbsp oyster sauce
1 tsp brown sugar
1 tbsp sesame oil
2 small red chillies, deseeded and sliced
200g/7oz firm tofu, diced
5cm/2in piece root ginger, peeled and grated
2 garlic cloves, crushed
150g/5½ oz shiitake mushrooms, sliced
6 spring onions, trimmed and chopped

Cover the noodles in boiling water and leave to soften for 5 minutes. Drain. In a bowl, mix together the soy sauce, oyster sauce and sugar. Heat the oil in a wok. Stir-fry the chillies, tofu, ginger and garlic for 2 minutes, then add the noodles, mushrooms, sauce mixture and spring onions. Toss and serve immediately.

FRIED SHIITAKE MUSHROOM SALAD

3 large handfuls mixed salad leaves
1 bunch watercress, trimmed
4 tbsp olive oil
450g/1lb shiitake mushrooms, stalks
   removed and caps sliced
8 garlic cloves, crushed
ground black pepper

Put the salad leaves and watercress in a bowl. Heat 3 tablespoons of the oil in a pan and sauté the mushrooms and garlic until tender. Add the contents of the pan to the salad with the remaining oil. Toss well, season with black pepper and serve.

STUFFED MUSHROOMS

4 large mushrooms
4 tbsp olive oil
4 spring onions, trimmed and chopped
1 red pepper, deseeded and finely chopped
2 small courgettes, chopped
8 green olives, pitted and chopped
2 tbsp porridge oats
1 tbsp chopped basil
1 tbsp soy sauce
salad leaves, to serve

Preheat the oven to 180°C/350°F/ gas mark 4. Remove the mushrooms' stalks. Heat the oil in a pan and gently fry the spring onions, pepper, courgettes, olives and oats for 3 minutes. Stir in the basil and soy sauce. Place the mushrooms on a baking tray and spoon the mixture over them. Bake for 15–20 minutes. Serve on a bed of salad.

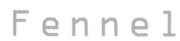

Fennel

Vitamins B1, B3, B5, B6, C, E, beta-carotene, biotin, folic acid; calcium, copper, iron, magnesium, phosphorus, potassium, selenium, zinc; ellagic acid; anethole, quercetin, rutin; carbohydrate; fibre

Part of the parsley family, the fennel plant and seeds have ancient healing properties and are also popular culinary ingredients. Used particularly in French and Italian cuisine, fennel boasts a host of anti-aging properties.

Fennel is well known for its anti-spasmodic, analgesic and diuretic properties. It can be used to ease digestive problems, combat fluid retention and reduce intestinal spasms. Because it aids the elimination of toxins through the urine, it is also a useful remedy for arthritis and gout. Its volatile oils have an antiseptic effect, and are considered particularly useful for combating urinary infections.

Rich in phytonutrients, including rutin, quercetin and anethole, fennel has been shown to reduce inflammatory conditions such as arthritis. Rutin strengthens blood capillaries, thereby improving poor circulation, while quercetin inhibits inflammatory conditions such as asthma. Anethole is anti-spasmodic, preventing the intestinal spasms often experienced by people with irritable bowel syndrome.

Fennel is also an excellent source of vitamin C, which is needed for the proper functioning of the immune system, to protect the brain and to avoid aging of the arteries. Fennel is fibre-rich and may help to reduce elevated cholesterol levels. In addition, it's a good source of folic acid, a vitamin that lowers the risk of heart disease.

SAUTÉED FENNEL

1 tbsp olive oil
2 fennel bulbs, trimmed and finely sliced
8 cloves garlic, crushed
ground black pepper
wholegrain bread and cheese, to serve

Heat the oil in a pan, add the fennel and garlic and gently fry until slightly soft. Season with black pepper. Serve as an accompaniment or with some wholegrain bread and cheese.

✦FENNEL MOUTHWASH *to protect teeth & gums*

½ tsp fennel seeds
½ tsp ground cloves
2 tbsp pure grain alcohol or good-quality vodka
250ml/9fl oz/1 cup distilled water
paper coffee filter

In a bowl, mix the spices into the alcohol. Cover and leave for 3 days, then pour through the coffee filter placed in a strainer. Add the water. Store in a sealed bottle for 6 weeks. Gargle with 1 tablespoon at a time, as a mouthwash.

✳FENNEL-SEED INFUSION
to cleanse & tone the skin

2 tsp fennel seeds, crushed
2 thyme sprigs, crumbled, or ½ tsp dried thyme
125ml/4fl oz/½ cup boiling water
juice of ½ lemon

In a bowl, combine the fennel seeds and thyme, and cover with the boiling water. Add the lemon juice and steep for 15 minutes. Strain, and when cold, store, covered, in a jar in the fridge. Dab evenly on the face and neck every morning with cotton wool, then rinse off with warm water.

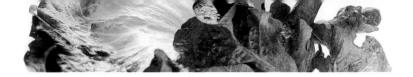

Lettuce

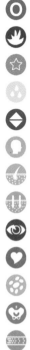

VITAMINS B1, B2, B3, B5, C, E, K, BETA-CAROTENE, BIOTIN, FOLIC ACID; CALCIUM, CHROMIUM, COPPER, IODINE, IRON, MAGNESIUM, MANGANESE, MOLYBDENUM, PHOSPHORUS, POTASSIUM, SELENIUM, SILICA, ZINC; FIBRE; PROTEIN; TRYPTOPHAN; LACTUCARIUM

A salad staple, lettuce helps to cleanse the blood, relax the nerves and eliminate excess fluid as well as providing vital nutrients for helping the body to make energy.

It looks insubstantial, but a lettuce leaf could be a powerful protector against one of the most frequent accidents that disable older people. Scientists have found that older women who eat lettuce every day have half as many hip fractures as those who eat it less than once a week. It's the vitamin K content that does so much good. Any kind of lettuce helps, but, as with other leafy foods, the darker the colour of the leaves, the more nutritional value the lettuce contains.

With its high potassium content, lettuce is also a mild diuretic, while its chlorophyll helps to detoxify the blood and liver. Other nutrients in lettuce include folic acid, important for preventing birth defects, and beta-carotene and vitamin C, two antioxidant vitamins, which help to bolster the immune system.

This leafy vegetable contains many minerals, including iron, calcium, magnesium and zinc, all of which help to generate energy. Equally important is the folic acid content – this B-vitamin protects the heart by converting a harmful chemical called homocysteine into benign substances. If not converted, homocysteine can directly damage blood vessels, greatly increasing the risk of heart attack and stroke.

Lettuce also contains a natural sedative that relaxes the nervous system and induces sleep.

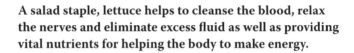

PEAS AND LETTUCE

55g/2oz butter
350g/12oz/2¼ cups peas
8 large cos lettuce leaves, cut into strips
4 tbsp stock or water
1 tsp ground black pepper

Melt the butter over a gentle heat and add the peas and lettuce. Add the stock or water and bring to the boil, then simmer, covered, for 5 minutes. Season with pepper and serve.

GREEN SALAD SUPREME

3 large handfuls mixed lettuce leaves
½ cucumber, sliced
100g/3½oz feta cheese, cubed
1 avocado, pitted, peeled and chopped
2 tbsp salad cress
2 tbsp chopped chives
2 tbsp olive oil
1 tbsp cider vinegar
salt and ground black pepper

Put all the ingredients in a large bowl, toss well and serve immediately.

CHEESY GRILLED LETTUCE

1 cos lettuce
1 tbsp olive oil
200g/7oz Camembert cheese
2 tsp balsamic vinegar

Preheat oven at 220°C/425°F/gas mark 7. Cut the lettuce lengthways into quarters, brush with the oil and grill for 2 minutes on each side. Arrange in a shallow ovenproof dish, top with thin slices of Camembert and drizzle with the vinegar. Bake for 5 minutes until the cheese is bubbling, then serve.

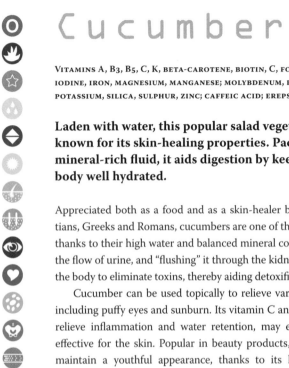

Cucumber

VITAMINS A, B3, B5, C, K, BETA-CAROTENE, BIOTIN, C, FOLIC ACID; CALCIUM,
IODINE, IRON, MAGNESIUM, MANGANESE; MOLYBDENUM, PHOSPHORUS,
POTASSIUM, SILICA, SULPHUR, ZINC; CAFFEIC ACID; EREPSIN; FIBRE

Laden with water, this popular salad vegetable is well known for its skin-healing properties. Packed with mineral-rich fluid, it aids digestion by keeping the body well hydrated.

Appreciated both as a food and as a skin-healer by the ancient Egyptians, Greeks and Romans, cucumbers are one of the best diuretic foods thanks to their high water and balanced mineral content. By promoting the flow of urine, and "flushing" it through the kidneys, cucumber helps the body to eliminate toxins, thereby aiding detoxification.

Cucumber can be used topically to relieve various skin afflictions, including puffy eyes and sunburn. Its vitamin C and caffeic acid, which relieve inflammation and water retention, may explain why it is so effective for the skin. Popular in beauty products, cucumber helps to maintain a youthful appearance, thanks to its hydrating and anti-inflammatory properties.

The rich fibre content of cucumbers keeps the digestive system moving and, unlike some other high-fibre foods, comes balanced with its own supply of fluid. Eating cucumbers can ease or prevent constipation, which is often exacerbated by not drinking enough water. It's helpful, too, if you've had diarrhoea, because as well as rehydrating, it replaces vital minerals. Cucumber is also a source of erepsin, an enzyme that helps the body to digest protein. Fresh cucumber juice can alleviate acid reflux and indigestion and is also useful for treating gum disease.

The minerals in cucumbers are clustered in the peel. The magnesium and potassium help to keep blood pressure in check. Cucumbers are a rich source of silica, needed for healthy skin, bone and connective tissue, and together with sulphur, this mineral promotes the growth of healthy hair and strong nails. Silica also plays a major role in preventing cardiovascular disease and osteoporosis.

GARDEN SALAD

100g/3½oz baby spinach leaves
1 cucumber, chopped
8 radishes, trimmed and thinly sliced
2 carrots, peeled and thinly sliced
1 spring onion, trimmed and chopped
2 tbsp chopped parsley
1 tbsp olive oil
juice of ½ lime

Combine the vegetables and parsley in a large bowl. Pour over the olive oil and lime juice, and toss well. Serve immediately.

CUCUMBER AND MINT SALAD

4 tbsp chopped mint, plus a few leaves
   to serve
1 large cucumber, chopped
2 celery sticks, trimmed and chopped
2 tsp white wine vinegar
8 tbsp/½ cup plain bio-yogurt

Mix together the chopped mint, cucumber and celery in a serving bowl. In a separate bowl, whisk the vinegar into the yogurt. Pour the dressing over the salad, add the mint leaves and serve.

*CUCUMBER LOTION to cleanse the skin

½ small cucumber
5 mint leaves
4 tbsp milk
2 drops grapefruit seed extract

Peel and chop the cucumber. Remove the mint leaves from their stalks and chop. Put both in a food processor with the milk and whizz until smooth. Pour the mixture into a saucepan and bring to the boil. Reduce the heat and simmer for 2 minutes, then allow to cool. Pour into a clean bottle and add the grapefruit seed extract. Store in the fridge and use within a week.

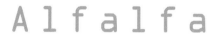

Alfalfa

VITAMINS A, B3, B5, C, D, E, K, BETA-CAROTENE, FOLIC ACID; CALCIUM, IRON, MAGNESIUM, MANGANESE, PHOSPHORUS, POTASSIUM, SILICA, SODIUM, ZINC; CHLOROPHYLL; SAPONINS; PROTEIN; FIBRE; ENZYMES

Highly digestible and containing huge amounts of antioxidants, alfalfa can be sprinkled on to any salad or added to any sandwich to boost your nutrient intake – and at virtually no calorie cost.

Long popular among health-food enthusiasts, alfalfa sprouts are packed with enzymes and easily digestible nutrients, which are unleashed during the sprouting process. Besides being a storehouse of amino acids, vitamins and minerals, alfalfa contains several phytochemicals that can protect against disease. Canavanine, an amino acid analogue, exerts anti-carcinogenic activity, while the plant oestrogens found in this food help to balance hormones. Other compounds abundant in alfalfa sprouts include saponins, which reduce cholesterol by binding to it so that the body can excrete it, and chlorophyll, a powerful blood-builder and detoxifying agent.

These sprouted seeds provide abundant amounts of vitamin A for the eyes, B-vitamins for the nervous system and brain power, vitamin C for immunity and eye health, and vitamin E for the skin and the heart. They are also high in calcium and phosphorus for the bones, iron to prevent anaemia, magnesium and potassium to lower the risk of heart disease, zinc to prevent premature hair loss, and silica to promote glowing skin, strong nails and glossy hair.

Alfalfa is one of the few sprouted seeds that is readily available in supermarkets. It will also significantly boost zinc intake, particularly when combined with chicory, to improve both liver and hormone function as well as promoting cellular growth and renewal.

Packed with nutrients, sprouts provide a burst of energy to see you through any form of exercise. Alfalfa contains a compound that inhibits fungal growth, an occasional by-product of sweaty environments. Rich in enzymes and fibre, alfalfa sprouts are easy to digest and contain very few calories, so they are useful for anyone trying to lose weight, too.

TOFU, AVOCADO AND ALFALFA POCKETS

200g/7oz smoked tofu, sliced

4 wholemeal pitta breads

2 large handfuls of alfalfa sprouts

2 avocados, pitted, peeled and sliced

2 tomatoes, sliced

12 pitted black olives, chopped

2 tbsp tahini

Grill the tofu slices on both sides. Warm the pittas briefly in an oven, then cut them along the top and stuff with the tofu, alfalfa, avocados, tomatoes and olives. Put the tahini and 6 tablespoons of water in a bowl and mix well. Spoon it over the pitta filling and serve

ALFALFA SALAD

4 large tomatoes

225g/8oz mixed salad leaves (such as lettuce, watercress and spinach)

115g/4oz/2 cups alfalfa sprouts

1 tsp white wine vinegar

2 tsp olive oil

1 spring onion, trimmed and chopped

1 garlic clove, crushed

salt and ground black pepper, to taste

Cut the tomatoes into wedges, and mix them with the salad leaves and alfalfa sprouts in a large bowl. For the dressing, mix together the remaining ingredients and pour over the salad just before serving.

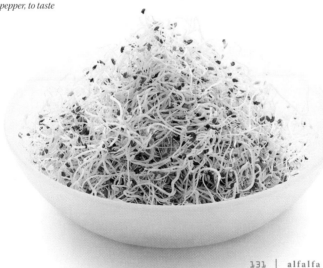

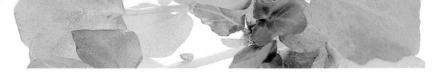

Watercress

Vitamins B1, B3, B5, B6, C, E, K, beta-carotene, biotin, folic acid; calcium, iodine, iron, magnesium, manganese, phosphorus, potassium, zinc; glucosinolates; fibre; protein

Packed with more than 15 vitamins and minerals, watercress has long enjoyed superfood status. This robustly flavoured salad leaf is a powerful immune-system stimulant.

Weight for weight, watercress contains more calcium than milk, more iron than spinach and as much vitamin C as oranges, making it an excellent food for the bones, blood and immune system. It is also a fabulous source of lutein and zeaxanthin – types of carotenoids that reduce the risk of eye disease. Watercress also possesses a unique compound called PEITC, which has not only been found to inhibit the growth of cancer, but is thought to kill existing cancerous cells as well. It also contains phenethyl isothiocyanate, a compound that helps the liver to detoxify and is particularly potent against lung cancer and bronchitis.

Watercress is rich in glucosinolates – plant chemicals that boost the activity of cancer-preventing enzymes. It contains the key antioxidant vitamins needed for a fully functioning immune system, along with vitamin B6, which enhances the action of phagocytes – white blood cells responsible for cleaning up waste matter. This vitamin also helps the release of bile from the gall bladder, which is important for the digestion of fat. It also helps to prevent memory loss.

A diuretic, watercress has expectorant and depurative properties, therefore easing inflammation, ulcers and boils and improving skin quality. It is also a good source of the mineral manganese, and iron, which both help the body to resist infections. Watercress is also a useful source of iodine, which is essential for the proper functioning of the thyroid.

STIR-FRIED WATERCRESS WITH ALMONDS AND GINGER

4 tbsp flaked almonds

2 tbsp sesame oil

450g/1lb watercress, chopped

5cm/2in piece root ginger, finely chopped

4 tbsp miso

4 tbsp rice vinegar

Heat a wok or pan and briefly dry-fry the almonds, then set aside. Add the oil to the wok and stir-fry the watercress and ginger for 3 minutes. Add the miso, rice vinegar and the almonds, stir well and serve immediately.

CREAMY WATERCRESS SOUP

55g/2oz butter

2 bunches watercress, chopped

1 onion, diced

25g/1oz/¼ cup plain flour

500ml/17fl oz/2 cups milk

455ml/16fl oz/scant 2 cups vegetable stock

6 tbsp single cream

Melt the butter in a pan and gently fry the watercress and onion for 3 minutes. Stir in the flour and cook for 1 minute. Slowly add the milk and then the stock, while stirring. Bring to the boil and stir until thickened. Cover and simmer for 30 minutes. Whizz the mixture in a blender, then add the cream and reheat gently without boiling. Serve.

WATERCRESS, CHICORY AND ORANGE SALAD

4 chicory

juice of 1 lemon

200g/7oz watercress, stalks discarded

4 oranges, peeled

2 carrots, peeled and grated

150ml/5fl oz/⅔ cup apple juice

salt and ground black pepper

Slice the chicory, place in a large salad bowl and squeeze over the lemon juice. Roughly chop the watercress and quarter the oranges. Combine them in the bowl with the remaining ingredients, season and toss well. Serve immediately.

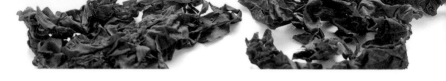

Seaweed

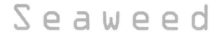

VITAMINS B1, B2, B3, B5, B6, B12, C, E, K, BETA-CAROTENE, FOLIC ACID; CAL-
CIUM, COPPER, IODINE, IRON, MAGNESIUM, MANGANESE, PHOSPHORUS, POTAS-
SIUM, SELENIUM, SODIUM, ZINC; LIGNANS; OMEGA-3 ESSENTIAL FATTY ACIDS;
COMPLEX CARBOHYDRATE, FIBRE; PROTEIN

Seaweed is a marine algae, the oldest form of life on the planet, and it contains a host of health-giving properties, particularly minerals. These gifts from the ocean could help to soothe away stress and put an end to insomnia by promoting peaceful sleep.

Seaweed, or sea vegetables, can be found both in salt water and in fresh-water lakes and seas. Best known for their use in Japanese cuisine, they offer an unrivalled range of nutrients that promote emotional health and keep the brain alert. They contain a wide range of minerals: magnesium helps to relieve stress-related symptoms such as heart palpitations; calcium helps to stabilize moods; and iron provides energy to the many people – especially young women – whose iron stores are low. The wide range of sea vegetables now available are rich in iodine, which supports metabolic and thyroid function. A slightly underactive thyroid, which is fairly common, especially among women, often causes depression and lethargy before any other signs lead to diagnosis.

Seaweed is among the foods credited with helping Japanese women to keep their legendary composure through life's changes. It contains phytonutrients called lignans, which work as a gentle form of hormone-replacement therapy. Eaten regularly, seaweed could help to reduce stress-inducing symptoms of the perimenopause, such as hot flushes. The plentiful nutrients found in sea vegetables could relieve sleepless-ness. The calming effects of magnesium, in particular, may counteract insomnia, as well as ease anxiety. Along with calcium, it can also prevent the leg cramps and restlessness that keep many women awake at night after the menopause.

Filled with mucilaginous gels that alkalinize the blood, seaweed can treat rheumatic complaints. It also helps to clear liver stagnation, treat-ing PMS, headaches and skin problems.

Agar-agar: Rich in trace minerals, agar-agar is used to soothe the digestive tract and relieve constipation. Its high fibre content helps to lower cholesterol and suppress the appetite, making it an ideal food for dieters. Its main culinary function is as a gelling agent.

Kombu: Laden with protein and minerals such as calcium, magnesium, potassium, iodine and iron, kombu improves the nutritional value of any meal. A substance in kombu called fucoidan has been found to make cancer cells self-destruct, and is now available as a nutritional supplement. Owing to kombu's excellent nutrient profile and cleansing abilities, it can offer relief in a range of health conditions from rheumatism, arthritis and high blood pressure to an under-active thyroid.

Nori: Used in sushi-making, this "fishy"-tasting seaweed has been cultivated in Japan for over a thousand years. An excellent source of protein, nori helps with growth and tissue repair, and its calcium and iron content nourishes the bones and blood. Particularly high in beta-carotene, nori may help to promote skin health, boost the immune system and slow down eye disease. It also contains vitamin B12, which is rarely found in the plant world, making it an ideal food for strict vegetarians.

Wakame: Traditionally added to miso soup, wakame is mild in flavour. It's an excellent source of potassium and may improve heart health by keeping high blood pressure in check. It's also an outstanding source of calcium, needed for bone maintenance, and magnesium for relieving stress and muscle tension. In Japan, wakame is used as a blood purifier and is also valued for its nourishing effect on the hair and skin.

Dulse: Full of potassium, which helps to relieve fluid retention, dulse is also the most iron-rich of the edible seaweeds, making it an excellent food for combating anaemia. Like most sea vegetables, it's high in iodine, which is needed to regulate the thyroid gland.

Hijiki: High in minerals, hijiki is thought to play a contributory role to the thick, shiny hair enjoyed by many Japanese people. It's a superb bone-builder, containing more calcium than any other sea vegetable, and it may help to prevent osteoporosis.

SEAWEED RICE

2 tbsp wakame
625ml/20fl oz/2½ cups warm water
½ onion, chopped
2 large garlic cloves, finely chopped
200g/7oz/1 cup brown rice

Rinse the wakame, and soak in the warm water for 5 minutes. Squeeze dry and chop. Save the water and heat 1 tablespoon in a pan. Simmer the onion gently for 2 minutes, stirring. Add all the other ingredients and the remaining water. Bring to the boil, then simmer for 35 minutes. Serve.

LAVER CAKES

450g/1lb laver, or rehydrated cooked nori, chopped
225g/8oz/1¾ cups rolled oats
1 tsp ground black pepper
3 tbsp oil
450g/1lb Portobello mushrooms

Mix together the laver, oatmeal and pepper in a bowl. Using your hands, shape into 12 balls and flatten slightly to make cakes. Heat 2 tablespoons of the oil and fry the cakes for 2–3 minutes. Brush the mushrooms with the remaining oil and grill until brown. Serve with the laver cakes.

WAKAME NOODLE BROTH

2 tbsp sesame oil
1 garlic clove, crushed
2 celery sticks, trimmed and chopped
1l/35fl oz/4 cups vegetable stock
1 tbsp miso
2 carrots, peeled and diced
8 strips wakame, chopped
50g/1¾oz dried noodles

Put all the ingredients (except the noodles) in a large pan, and bring to the boil, stirring until the miso has dissolved. Simmer, covered, for 30 minutes. Add the noodles and cook for a further few minutes until they are cooked through. Serve immediately.

REAL FRUIT JELLY

400g/14oz soft fruit, chopped (such as
   peaches, strawberries, grapes)
600ml/21fl oz/2⅓ cups white grape juice
4 tbsp agar-agar flakes

Place the chopped fruit in a large
heatproof glass bowl and set aside.
Put the grape juice and agar-agar in a
pan, bring to the boil and simmer for
a few minutes while stirring, until the
agar-agar has dissolved. Pour the
liquid over the fruit and leave to cool.
Once set, store in the fridge.

MISO SOUP

4 tbsp chopped dulse
2 tbsp wakame
2.5cm/1in piece root ginger, finely chopped
115g/4oz firm tofu, cut into cubes
3 tbsp miso

Pour 1.2l/44fl oz/5 cups water into a
pan and add the seaweeds, ginger and
tofu. Bring to the boil and simmer for
5 minutes. Stir in the miso, heat for 2
minutes and serve.

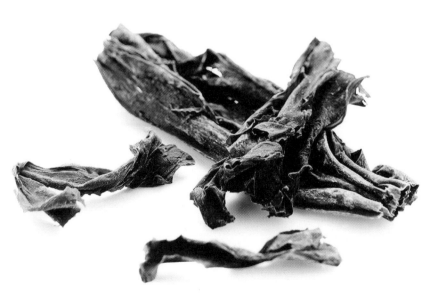

CANNELLINI KOMBU BEAN POT

200g/7oz/1 cup dried cannellini beans
1 strip dried kombu
½ leek, trimmed and chopped
½ red pepper, deseeded and chopped
200g/7oz spinach, chopped

Soak the beans overnight in plenty of cold water. Next day, drain, place in a pan and cover with 1l/35fl oz/ 4 cups water. Add the kombu, then bring to the boil and simmer, covered, for about 2 hours until the beans are soft. Add the leek, red pepper and spinach, and cook for a further 15 minutes. Mix well and serve.

KOMBU TOMATO STOCK

1 strip dried kombu
6 sun-dried tomatoes

Soak the kombu and tomatoes in 1l/35fl oz/4 cups water for 30 minutes, then bring to the boil and simmer for 5 minutes. Remove the kombu and tomatoes. Use the liquid for any recipe that calls for stock. The kombu can be reused to make more stock or added to beans or casseroles during cooking to enhance the flavour.

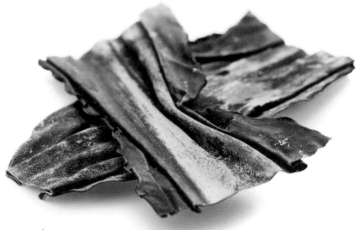

NORI POTATO FRITTERS

2 large potatoes, peeled and coarsely
  grated
1 onion, finely chopped
4 eggs
5 tbsp nori flakes
1 tbsp ground mustard seeds
olive oil, for shallow frying

Using your hands, squeeze as much of the juice from the grated potatoes as possible, then put them in a bowl and mix them with the onion, eggs, nori and mustard seeds. Warm the oil in a frying pan, adding the mixture when the oil is hot. Flatten each fritter with a fork and cook on both sides for a few minutes until golden.

SEA SALAD

3 tbsp dulse, rinsed
2 handfuls mixed salad leaves
½ cucumber, peeled and chopped
1 spring onion, trimmed and chopped
2 tbsp sesame oil
1 tbsp rice vinegar
1 tbsp sesame seeds

Soak the dulse in water for about 3 minutes, then drain and cut it into pieces with scissors. Put it in a large bowl along with the salad leaves, cucumber and spring onion. Add the sesame oil and rice vinegar, toss well and serve sprinkled with the sesame seeds.

SCRAMBLED EGGS WITH HIJIKI

2 heaped tbsp hijiki
1 tbsp olive oil
4 eggs
6 cherry tomatoes, sliced
2 tbsp finely chopped chives
1 tsp ground mustard seeds
1 garlic clove, crushed
salt and ground black pepper

Soak the hijiki in water for 15 minutes, then drain and sauté in the oil in a frying pan for about 8 minutes. Meanwhile, beat the eggs in a bowl and add the remaining ingredients. Pour the mixture over the hijiki and cook, stirring frequently, until the eggs have thickened but are still soft.

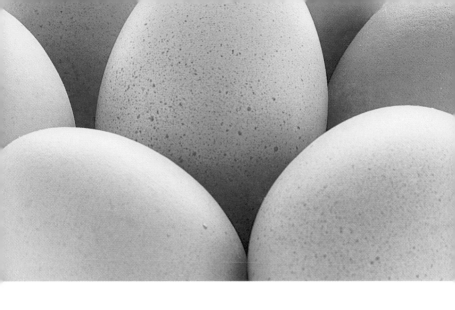

CRAMMED WITH PROTEIN,
THE BUILDING BLOCK
FOR OUR BONES, TISSUES
AND TEETH, MEAT AND
DAIRY PRODUCTS KEEP US
STRONG AND HEALTHY

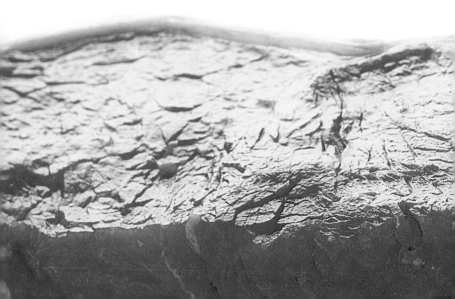

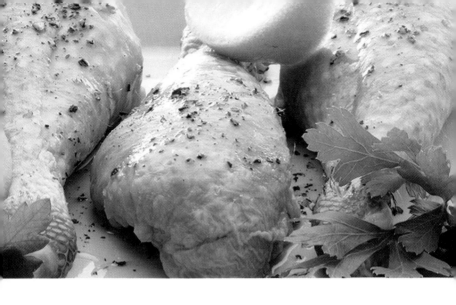

03 | wonder
MEAT & DAIRY

Lamb

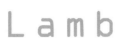

VITAMINS B1, B2, B3, B6, B12; IRON, PHOSPHORUS, SELENIUM, SULPHUR, ZINC; PROTEIN

A staple of many cuisines, lamb has valuable nutritious properties. Lean lamb is an excellent source of protein and easily absorbed iron.

Like other red meat, lamb is rich in protein, as well as being an excellent source of two vital minerals: iron and zinc. Iron helps to boost the oxygen-carrying capability of blood, preventing anaemia and fatigue from setting in, while zinc is necessary for optimum functioning of the immune system, helping to fight colds, infections and other invaders. According to the Chinese, eating lamb improves circulation, overcomes coldness and may even treat post-natal depression.

Lamb is a rich source of B-vitamins, including vitamin B3, which is thought to stave off age-related memory problems, and vitamin B12, which helps in the production of red blood cells and plays an important role in cell metabolism. The meat is also rich in easily absorbed iron, which is fundamental for preventing anaemia. The selenium in lamb protects the eyes from disease and the heart from muscle damage.

The high protein content in lamb, which is necessary to repair aging cells, helps to suppress the appetite for longer and prolongs satiety more than foods high in carbohydrate or fat. Lamb is also rich in sulphur, a mineral good for the hair and nails, and a key component of chondroitin sulphate, a complex molecule that gives cartilage the elastic, sponge-like quality that joints need to act as shock absorbers between the bones.

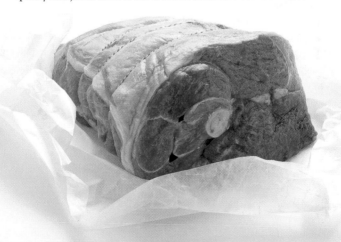

LAMB KOFTA

450g/1lb finely minced lamb
1 large onion, grated
1 tsp salt
30g/1oz/1 cup finely chopped parsley
¼ tsp black pepper
1 tsp ground allspice

Combine the ingredients and chill for 1 hour. Divide and shape into 8 balls, then thread the balls onto skewers. Cook under the grill until browned on all sides.

LAMB SHANKS IN TOMATO-ORANGE SAUCE

oil, for greasing
4 lamb shanks
450g/1lb/1¾ cups tinned, chopped
   tomatoes
250ml/9fl oz/1 cup water
1 tbsp crushed garlic
juice and grated zest of 1 orange
2 tbsp mint, finely chopped

Lightly grease a large pan. Add the lamb and cook, turning as needed, for 10 minutes or until lightly browned on all sides. Add the tomatoes, water, garlic, orange juice and zest to the pan. Cover and simmer for 2–3 hours or until the meat is tender. Stir in the mint, and serve.

LAMB AND POTATO TRAYBAKE

800g/1lb 2oz new potatoes
8 bay leaves
2 red onions, sliced
2 tbsp olive oil
juice of 1 lemon
8 lamb loin chops
1 handful mint, chopped

Preheat the oven to 220°C/425°F/gas mark 7. Put the potatoes, bay leaves and onions on a baking tray. Sprinkle with a little olive oil and the lemon juice, cover with foil and roast for 40 minutes. In a frying pan, brown the chops on both sides in the remaining oil. Remove the foil, add the chops and mint, and roast for a further 15 minutes.

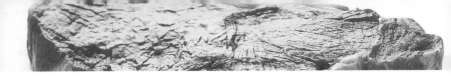

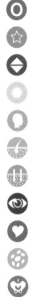

Beef

VITAMINS B1, B2, B3, B5, B6, B12; IRON, SULPHUR, ZINC; CONJUGATED LINOLEIC ACID; PROTEIN

A popular meat for millennia in many ancient cultures, beef is a flavourful meat with many therapeutic attributes. It is particularly high in iron, which boosts the oxygen level in the blood.

Rich in protein, beef is also full of B-complex vitamins, including B1, B2, B3, B5 and B6, which collectively help to protect against chronic fatigue syndrome, weak digestion, eye disease, depression and mood swings. It is also an excellent source of vitamin B12, which helps to prevent fatigue and protect against memory loss.

Beef is loaded with iron, which is needed for the production of red blood cells and staves off conditions such as anaemia. Full of zinc to boost immunity and aid the healing of wounds, this tasty red meat also contains sulphur, which we need to maintain youthful hair and nails.

According to the Chinese, eating beef lifts body metabolism, treats hypoglycaemia and strengthens the bones. Organic beef is free from pesticides and contains conjugated linoleic acid (CLA), a fatty acid that has cancer-fighting properties and helps people trying to lose weight by stimulating the conversion of stored fat in the body into energy.

PEPPER STEAKS

4 beef fillet steaks

2 tbsp olive oil

6 tbsp assorted cracked peppercorns

2 garlic cloves, crushed

40g/1½oz butter

salt and ground black pepper

Coat the steaks with the olive oil. Press down on the peppercorns with a knife, then press them into the steaks. Coat the steaks thoroughly with the crushed garlic. Melt the butter in a large frying pan. Cook the steaks over a medium heat for 3–4 minutes on each side. Season to taste with salt and pepper.

Duck

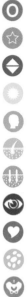

VITAMINS B1, B2, B3, B6, B12; COPPER, IRON, PHOSPHORUS, SELENIUM, ZINC; PROTEIN

Duck is delicious roasted or stir-fried and is an excellent source of the stress-busting vitamin B2 and an energy-rich way for athletes to hit their daily protein target.

Ducks were first domesticated in China, where they are appreciated for their eggs. Today, duck is a popular and uniquely flavoursome variety of poultry as well as a wonderful source of immunity-boosting nutrients.

Although duck has a reputation as a fat-laden meat, its saturated fat content is five times lower when all the skin is removed – in fact, a skinless duck breast is leaner than a skinless chicken breast. Duck meat provides plenty of the protein and iron needed to repair body tissue and build new red blood cells, as well as phosphorus, necessary for strong bones. Its copper content is needed for wound-healing and for the formation of collagen and elastin, which keep the skin looking and feeling youthful, while its selenium helps to neutralize the aging effects of free radicals on the body.

Duck is high in a host of B-vitamins, which help to fight fatigue, regulate metabolism and lift the mood. Eating duck will also help you to combat stress, as it contains the vitamin B2 and aids the production of infection-fighting immune cells.

DUCK STIR-FRY

1 red onion, finely chopped

1 tbsp sesame oil

2 tbsp soy sauce

4 Mallard duck breasts, skinned and cut into strips

2 carrots, peeled and cut into batons

400g/14oz mung bean sprouts

juice and grated zest of 1 orange

Fry the onion in a wok in the oil and soy sauce. Add the duck breast strips and carrots and fry for 5 minutes. Then, add the bean sprouts and orange juice and zest, and cook for a further minute.

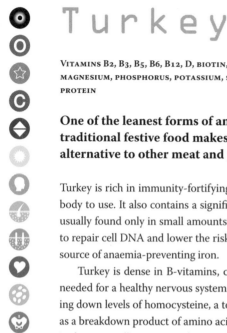

Turkey

Vitamins B2, B3, B5, B6, B12, D, biotin, folic acid; calcium, iodine, iron, magnesium, phosphorus, potassium, selenium, tryptophan; zinc; protein

One of the leanest forms of animal protein, this traditional festive food makes a healthier everyday alternative to other meat and poultry.

Turkey is rich in immunity-fortifying zinc in a form that is easy for the body to use. It also contains a significant amount of selenium, which is usually found only in small amounts in many foods. This mineral helps to repair cell DNA and lower the risk of cancer. The meat is also a good source of anaemia-preventing iron.

Turkey is dense in B-vitamins, crucial for normal metabolism and needed for a healthy nervous system. They are also important for keeping down levels of homocysteine, a toxic substance in the blood formed as a breakdown product of amino acids and linked with heart disease. It is also an excellent source of tryptophan, which plays an important role in boosting immunity, as well as helping in the treatment of insomnia.

Research shows that turkey contains one of the highest concentrations of muscle-building dipeptides. In tests, athletes who regularly ate 140g/5oz portions of turkey breast meat showed an increase of 40 per cent in muscle concentration. Their performance improved greatly, especially for runners, rowers, cyclists and speed skaters.

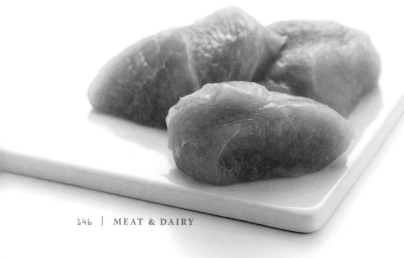

DELUXE TURKEY SANDWICH *serves 1*

½ avocado
2 slices wholegrain bread
fresh spinach leaves
2 cooked turkey slices
1 spring onion, trimmed and finely
  chopped
1 tomato, sliced
1 tsp wholegrain mustard (optional)

Scoop out the avocado flesh and spread over the bread like butter. Layer the spinach and turkey slices on one slice and top with the spring onion, tomato, and mustard, if desired. Sandwich together and eat immediately.

TURKEY AND PEPPER BURRITOS

2 turkey breasts, diced
1 red onion, chopped
1 red pepper, deseeded and cut into strips
1 tbsp sunflower oil
6 tbsp salsa
4 large flour tortillas
1 handful grated cheese

Preheat the oven to180°C/350°F/gas mark 4. Stir-fry the turkey, onion and pepper in the oil for 5–6 minutes. Add the salsa and heat through. Warm the tortillas in the oven, then place the mixture in the centre of each. Roll them up and place them seam-side down on a baking tray and top with cheese. Bake for 10–12 minutes, then serve.

TURKEY SCHNITZEL

4 turkey breasts, about 175g/6oz each,
  flattened
3 tbsp plain flour
1 large egg, beaten
115g/4oz/4 cups cornflakes, finely crushed
green salad, to serve

Preheat the oven to180°C/350°F/gas mark 4. Coat the turkey pieces lightly in the flour. Dip them in the egg and then coat in the cornflakes. Place on a baking tray and bake for 25 minutes, until the juices run clear. Serve with a green salad.

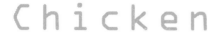

Chicken

VITAMINS A, B2, B3, B6, B12, K; IRON, MAGNESIUM, PHOSPHORUS, POTASSIUM, SELENIUM, SODIUM, ZINC; LYSINE; TRYPTOPHAN; PROTEIN

This hugely versatile and popular meat has a host of health-boosting properties. Dating back to the ancient Egyptians in the fourteenth century BC, chicken has become an everyday food full of goodness.

A useful source of protein, and low fat if the skin is removed, chicken contributes to the growth and repair of all the body's cells. The meat is a good source of B-complex vitamins, which also help to regulate the metabolism, and is rich in absorbable iron and zinc – with twice as much in the dark meat as in the breast – so fighting anaemia and boosting immunity, while the breast is particularly high in vitamin B6, which protects the heart and fights pre-menstrual syndrome (PMS). Chicken's vitamin B3 and B6 content also help to maintain a healthy nervous system and work together to make the most of food's energizing potential.

Chicken contains magnesium to help reduce the risk of cramps during exercise, and potassium to balance the fluid levels in the body, as well as selenium, which helps to prevent wrinkles and keep the hair glossy, and zinc to bolster immunity. Zinc is also known to have energy-boosting properties. In addition, chicken has the anti-viral amino acid lysine, helpful for suppressing the cold-sore virus.

Another nutrient found in chicken is tryptophan, an essential amino acid that helps to control the brain's serotonin levels, which are linked to appetite and mood. Chicken promotes circulation and invigorates the kidneys, thus treating diarrhoea and oedema. Made into a soup, chicken is known to be soothing and restorative. Chicken soup is an effective remedy for colds and infections of the upper respiratory tract.

A high intake of saturated fats increases the risk of heart disease and piles on the kilos/pounds, significantly slowing an athlete down. Lean meat is a top choice for anyone taking regular exercise, and chicken is one of the leanest, as long as you resist eating the skin. Always buy organic chicken, which is now widely available, as it offers all the nutritional benefits without the possible drug residues.

ZESTY CHICKEN CASSEROLE

3 tbsp olive oil

2 onions, sliced

8 skinless chicken thighs

1 tbsp plain flour, seasoned with a little
    salt and pepper

300ml/10½fl oz/scant 1¼ cups
    vegetable stock

grated zest of 1 orange and juice of 2 oranges

150ml/5fl oz/scant ⅔ cup white wine

5 Portobello mushrooms, sliced

rice, to serve

Heat 2 tablespoons of olive oil in a
frying pan, add the onions and fry
for 10 minutes. Transfer to a plate.
Toss the chicken in the flour, heat the
remaining oil, add the chicken and
fry until browned. Add the bouillon,
onions, orange juice and zest, and
white wine. Bring to the boil, reduce
heat, cover and simmer for 25
minutes. Stir in the mushrooms and
cook for 5 minutes. Serve with rice.

GRANDMA'S CHICKEN SOUP

2¼l/80fl oz/9 cups chicken broth

6 garlic cloves, minced

2.5cm/1in piece root ginger, peeled and cut
    into 2 or 3 chunks

225g/8oz skinless, boneless chicken
    breasts, cubed

4 spring onions, trimmed and chopped

Bring the broth, garlic and ginger to
the boil in a pan, then simmer for
10 minutes. Add the chicken and
cook for 5–7 minutes. Discard the
ginger. Top with the onions to serve.

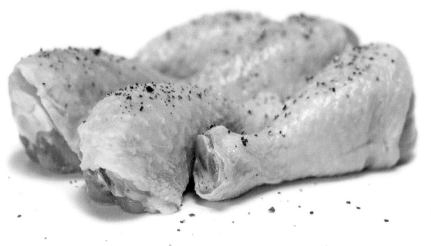

SWEET AND SOUR CHICKEN DRUMSTICKS

8 chicken drumsticks, skinned

4 tbsp clear honey

2 tbsp sesame oil

90ml/3fl oz/⅓ cup soy sauce

4 tbsp lemon juice

4 tsp coarsegrain mustard

Preheat the oven to 200°C/400°F/gas mark 6. Put the drumsticks in an ovenproof dish and pierce with a fork. Mix the honey, sesame oil, soy sauce, lemon juice and mustard and pour over the chicken. Cook for 25–30 minutes. Serve hot or cold.

EASY MARINATED CHICKEN

3 tbsp soy sauce

3 tbsp rice wine or sherry

1 tsp sugar

2 cloves garlic, crushed

450g/1lb chicken breasts, cut into
  bite-sized pieces

Mix together the soy sauce, rice wine, sugar and garlic. Place the chicken in a dish, pour over the marinade, cover and place in a cool place for 2 hours.

BALSAMIC BARBECUE CHICKEN

6 tbsp balsamic vinegar

2 tbsp sunflower oil

1 tsp Dijon mustard

1 tsp clear honey

½ tsp salt

1 tsp ground black pepper

8 large chicken drumsticks

In a bowl, mix the vinegar, oil, mustard and honey, and season. Coat the drumsticks, and chill in a shallow dish for 2 hours. Grill on a barbecue for 15–20 minutes, turning every 5 minutes until cooked through and the juices run clear, then serve.

Bio-yogurt

VITAMINS A, B2, B3, B5, B12, C, D, BIOTIN, FOLIC ACID; CALCIUM, IODINE, IRON, MAGNESIUM, MOLYBDENUM, PHOSPHORUS, POTASSIUM, SELENIUM, SODIUM, ZINC; PROTEIN; BACTERIA CULTURES

Also known as live or probiotic yogurt, bio-yogurt is an immune-system saviour, positively brimming with "friendly" bacteria and many health-promoting nutrients.

Bio-yogurt contains health-boosting lactobacillus and bifida bacteria. A healthy gut should be teeming with these, but stress, antibiotics and poor diet can allow "unfriendly" bacteria to take over. Eating one pot of live yogurt a day can help to redress the balance, aiding the body to fight off infections, as well as allowing the gut to absorb other immunity-boosting nutrients efficiently. Yogurt also stimulates the production of antiviral agents, which enhance immune response and help to ward off cancer.

Live yogurt can help to prevent constipation and alleviate the bloating, gas and vaginal thrush often caused by an overgrowth of candida yeast, which produces itching, burning and other uncomfortable symptoms. It can also avert antibiotic-related diarrhoea and keep invading organisms in check, and it is thought to offer some relief from stomach ulcers. Some studies have found that the probiotics present in yogurt produce enzymes that are absorbed directly through the gut wall, which further strengthens the body's immune defences.

Bio-yogurt has a high calcium content, as well as traces of vitamin D, which help us to absorb calcium. It also contains other bone-building minerals, such as magnesium and phosphorus. Eating it regularly reduces the risk of developing the bone-thinning condition, osteoporosis.

YOGURT WITH NUTS AND HONEY

400g/14oz/1½ cups plain bio-yogurt
1 handful walnut halves
4 tbsp clear honey
4 tbsp almonds

Mix the yogurt with the walnuts in a bowl. Drizzle the honey in a spiral around the top. Sprinkle with the almonds, and serve.

APPLE AND SEED YOGURT *serves 1*

200g/7oz/heaped ¾ cup plain bio-yogurt
2 tbsp sunflower seeds
1 green apple, cored and deseeded

Chop the apple into bite-sized chunks and place in a small bowl. Spoon the yogurt over the top, then sprinkle on the seeds and eat immediately. Can be enjoyed as a breakfast or as a snack at any time.

*YOGURT AND EVENING PRIMROSE FACE MASK
for revitalizing & replenishing tired skin

2 capsules evening primrose oil
2 capsules vitamin E oil
3 tbsp plain bio-yogurt
1 tsp clear honey
25g/1oz potato flour

Extract the oil from the capsules and combine it in a bowl with the other ingredients. Add extra flour to achieve the desired consistency, if necessary. Apply the mask evenly to the face and leave for approximately 20 minutes. Wash off with water and pat dry. Repeat the process each evening, as desired.

LASSI

250g/9oz/1 cup plain bio-yogurt
1 tsp cumin seeds
½ tsp salt
½ tsp finely chopped mint

Put all the ingredients and 625ml/ 21fl oz/2½ cups cold water in a blender and whizz for a few seconds, until well mixed. Serve cold.

AMBROSIA FRUIT SALAD *serves 2*

2 tbsp flaked almonds
2 tbsp flaked coconut
200g/7oz tin pineapple chunks, drained
1 banana, chopped
200g/7oz/1 cup cherries, pitted
6 tbsp bio-yogurt
2 tbsp pure maple syrup
1 tsp ground cinnamon
½ tsp ground nutmeg

Toast the almonds and coconut in a dry pan for a few minutes, then transfer to a bowl and leave to cool. Add the fruit and yogurt and mix together so that all the ingredients are well combined. Spoon into individual dessert bowls, top with the maple syrup, cinnamon and nutmeg, and serve.

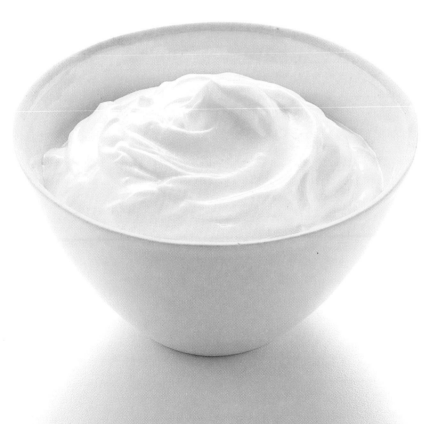

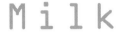

Milk

VITAMINS A, B2, B12, D, E, K; CALCIUM, IODINE, PHOSPHORUS, POTASSIUM; OMEGA-3 FATTY ACIDS; PROTEIN

Soothing and comforting, milk provides liquid nutrition helpful in preventing and treating a great many conditions. Best known for its calcium content, it helps to strengthen bones and fight off heart disease.

Milk is a first-class protein, providing building blocks that are especially useful in a child's diet. The abundance of calcium in milk gives it the ability to strengthen bones and to help to stave off osteoporosis. Studies have also shown that calcium may help to reduce blood pressure as well as lower cholesterol levels. Its potassium content is key in fighting heart disease and may prevent strokes. It may also contain substances that reduce the liver's production of cholesterol and lower blood pressure.

A good source of vitamin B12, which combats memory loss, hearing problems and fatigue, milk also contains vitamin B2, which is known to promote healthy skin and good vision. Another of its nutrients, the antioxidant vitamin E, also benefits the skin and eyes, as well as boosting the immune system. Skimmed milk is also believed to have anti-carcinogenic properties.

Many women become irritable, forgetful or depressed just before a period starts – the well-known symptoms of premenstrual syndrome (PMS). A glass of milk could be the simplest remedy, as it contains many nutrients that can lift and stabilize mood. It's rich in calcium and vitamin D, which together have been found to reduce or even prevent PMS symptoms. Cold milk can also be useful when you need to stay awake, because it triggers the brain's production of dopamine and noradrenaline, two substances that keep you alert.

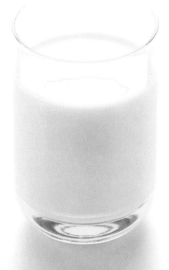

As with other animal foods, it's best to buy organic milk. This has been found to contain up to 70 per cent more omega-3 oils than ordinary milk, helping the brain to function at optimal efficiency.

Studies show that drinking chocolate milk improves endurance more than conventional carbohydrate-only sports drinks, because it contains the ideal ratio of carbohydrates to protein to help refuel tired muscles. Try a home-made milkshake, a smoothie or a cup of cocoa within two hours of exercise. The body converts these post-exercise calories into glycogen to deliver carbohydrate straight to fuel-depleted muscles.

*MILK AND HONEY BATH LOTION
to nourish the skin

2 eggs
3 tbsp carrier oil
150ml/5fl oz/⅔ cup milk
2 tsp clear honey
2 tsp shampoo
1 tbsp vodka

In a bowl, beat together the eggs and oil. Add the other ingredients, mix and pour into a glass bottle. Add 2–3 tablespoons to bath water. Keep the remaining lotion chilled and use within 3–4 days.

BEDTIME MILK serves 2

500ml/17fl oz/2 cups milk
a tiny pinch saffron
2 tbsp clear honey
1 tsp ground nutmeg
½ tsp ground cinnamon

Gently heat the milk, saffron and honey in a pan, stirring until the honey is dissolved. Pour into cups, sprinkle over the spices and serve.

CEREAL SOOTHER

350g/12oz wholegrain breakfast cereal
4 tbsp sunflower seeds
2 bananas, sliced
250ml/9fl oz/1 cup skimmed or
   semi-skimmed milk

Mix together the cereal and the seeds in a bowl. Divide between four bowls, top with the bananas and pour the milk over the top. Serve.

Egg

Vitamins A, B2, B3, B5, B6, B12, D, E, K, biotin, choline, folic acid, lutein, zeaxanthin; calcium, chromium, copper, iodine, iron, lecithin, magnesium, manganese, molybdenum, phosphorus, potassium, selenium, sodium, zinc; omega-3 essential fatty acids; protein

The perfect complete protein, these little capsules of nutrition are an excellent low-fat, slow-release energy food, stabilizing blood-sugar levels and keeping hunger pangs at bay. Low in fat and extremely versatile, eggs contain all the essential amino acids needed for peak fitness, staving off aging and boosting brain power.

Eggs are a superb source of B-vitamins, zinc, iron and phospholipids – fats required for cell membranes and a healthy brain. They're also one of the few non-meat sources of vitamin A, which supports vision; vitamin D, which we need for healthy bones; and B12, which aids many of the body's processes. The vitamin E contained in eggs is a powerful antioxidant, which thins the blood, benefits the heart and fights harmful free radicals. They also contain omega-3 fats and a B-vitamin called choline, both of which are required for normal brain function, and lutein, which can help to reduce the risk of eye disease. Moreover, eggs are rich in vitamin K, which helps to heal bruises and minor sports injuries by ensuring that blood is able to clot normally, so it could also reduce the danger of blood clots in arteries. In addition, eggs are a valuable source of selenium, which rejuvenates the immune system and protects the heart.

Low in saturated fats and high in protein, eggs have been shown by research to improve brain function. It is thought that their high lecithin content not only enhances the memory and the ability to concentrate but also promotes a healthy emotional state. Egg yolk is the richest known source of choline, the B-vitamin that makes up cell membranes, helping the body to convert fats to acetylcholine, an important memory molecule needed in the brain.

Eggs are a concentrated source of muscle-building amino acids and other body-building nutrients. Their high zinc content boosts immunity and is beneficial for liver function as well as tissue repair and healing. It is also vital for the production of collagen, which is needed for healthy, youthful skin. Because eggs contain all eight essential amino acids, thus helping to make up the building blocks for the entire body, they benefit everything from skin to hair, and bones to muscles.

Many of us worry about the apparently high cholesterol content of eggs, but studies suggest this may be unfounded as the cholesterol in eggs doesn't circulate in the blood. In fact, of the 5g of fat contained in an egg, most is monounsaturated, which is the type that helps to lower the risk of heart disease. The nutritional value of eggs has been found to vary, so it is best to choose the organic free-range variety, which contain more vitamins and good fats than eggs laid by battery hens.

✳ EGG YOLK MASK *to nourish dry skin*

1 tbsp clear honey
1 large egg yolk
1 tsp potato flour

In a bowl, combine the honey, egg yolk and potato flour, stirring to create a fine paste. Apply evenly to the face and neck and leave for about 20 minutes. Rinse off with cotton wool and water. Pat dry. Repeat 2 or 3 times a week, making a fresh mask for each treatment.

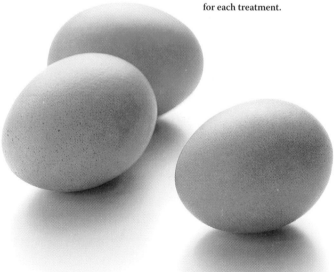

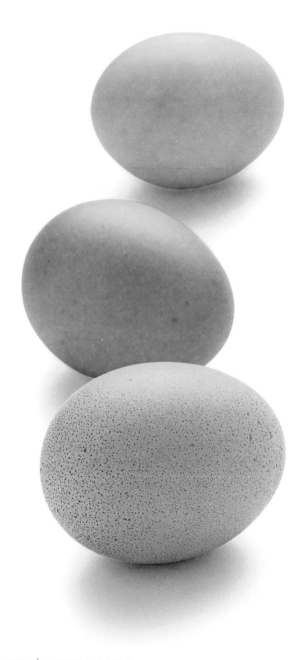

SMOKED SALMON WITH SCRAMBLED EGGS

6 eggs

salt and ground black pepper

1 tsp olive oil

85g/3oz smoked salmon

4 tbsp chopped dill or chives

lemon wedges, to garnish

Beat the eggs with some salt and pepper and heat in a pan with the oil, stirring all the time until just cooked. Pile on plates with the smoked salmon, sprinkle over the herbs and garnish with lemon wedges and more black pepper.

LEEK AND PEPPER OMELETTE

1 tbsp groundnut oil

1 leek, trimmed and finely chopped

1 sweet pepper, deseeded and diced

4 eggs

salt and ground black pepper

Heat the oil and gently fry the leek for 2–3 minutes until half cooked. Add the sweet pepper and cook for 2 minutes. Remove the vegetables with a slotted spoon and set aside. Beat the eggs in a bowl and add 2 tablespoons cold water. Season and pour the mixture into the pan. Add the vegetables and cook for around 5 minutes until the egg is set.

POTATO FRITTATA

450g/1lb potatoes, peeled and diced

1 tbsp olive oil

4 eggs, beaten

1 tbsp soy sauce

1 large handful chopped parsley

ground black pepper to taste

Steam the potatoes for 15 minutes, then transfer to the pan oiled with the olive oil. Mix together the remaining ingredients and pour them over the potatoes. Cook gently for 3–4 minutes. Once the underside is done, place under a grill and cook until golden and set.

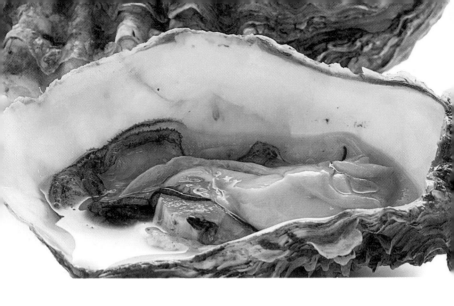

FROM SIMPLE TUNA
TO LUXURIOUS OYSTERS,
FISH AND SEAFOOD OFFER
A WEALTH OF BENEFITS
IN TANTALIZING TASTES
AND TEXTURES

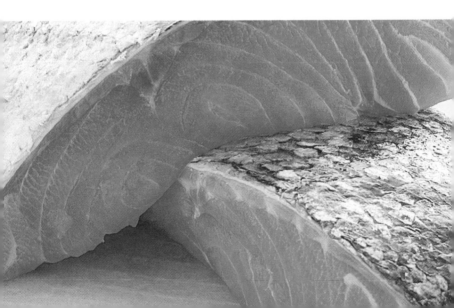

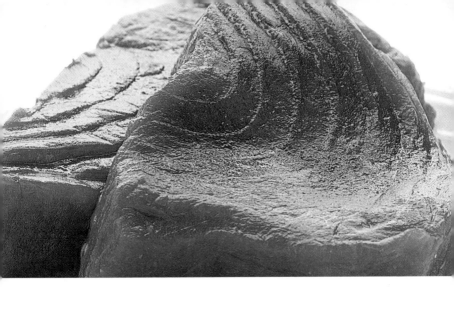

04 | **wonder FISH**

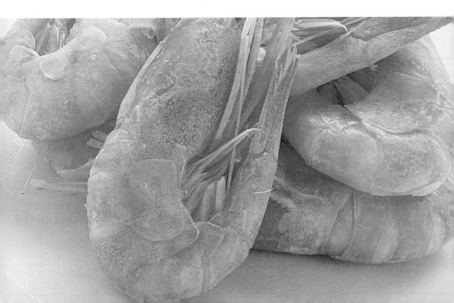

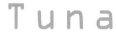

Tuna

VITAMINS B1, B3, B6, B12, D, E; IODINE, MAGNESIUM, PHOSPHORUS,
POTASSIUM, SELENIUM, SODIUM; OMEGA-3 FATTY ACIDS; PROTEIN; TRYPTOPHAN

A member of the mackerel family, tuna is rich in healthy oils and immunity-boosting minerals.

Popular sources of protein, such as meat and hard cheese, are often high in fat. Yet high-protein foods keep you going longer before flagging energy levels send you in search of a snack. Tuna is an excellent high-protein, low-fat option, providing more protein than even the healthiest meat. Lean sources of protein are key for anyone who's physically active, as they prevent slumps in energy without sending calorie intake soaring. The best choices are albacore, skipjack or yellowfin tuna.

Like other oily fish, fresh tuna is exceptionally rich in omega-3 fatty acids, which play an important role in energy production and helping to burn excess fat. Among their many other benefits, omega-3s stimulate the production of leptin, a hormone that controls the appetite. Essential fatty acids can help to prevent heart disease, cancer and depression and support the immune system. They are also anti-inflammatory, calming conditions such as rheumatoid arthritis and eczema.

Tuna contains vitamin E and selenium, which are needed for the production of disease-fighting antibodies, and many B-vitamins, which boost energy levels.

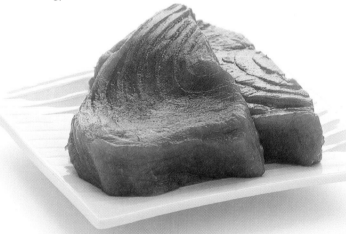

TUNA NIÇOISE

juice of 1 lemon
½ tsp salt
1 tsp Dijon mustard
5 tbsp olive oil
a pinch of ground black pepper
4 fresh tuna steaks
4 potatoes, cooked and sliced
115g/4oz green beans, cooked
115g/4oz mixed salad leaves
4 tomatoes, cut into segments
1 handful black olives

Whisk together the lemon juice, salt, mustard, olive oil and black pepper. Place the tuna steaks on a large plate and coat in the vinaigrette mixture. Chill for 1 hour, then grill for 4–6 minutes. Combine all the vegetables in a large salad bowl and drizzle over the remaining vinaigrette. Top with the tuna steaks and serve.

BAKED TUNA

4 fresh tuna steaks
black pepper, to taste
3 tbsp olive oil
2 onions, chopped
125ml/4fl oz/½ cup dry white wine
4 tomatoes, chopped

Preheat the oven to 220°C/425°F/gas mark 7. Put the tuna in an ovenproof dish and rub with pepper and 1 table-spoon of the oil. Heat the remaining oil in a frying pan and sauté the onions for 3–5 minutes. Add the wine and tomatoes, and bring to the boil. Pour over the tuna and bake for 15 minutes, until the tuna is cooked through. Serve.

TUNA WITH SALSA

4 fresh tuna steaks
2 tomatoes, chopped
2 red onions, finely diced
2 tbsp finely cut chives
1 tbsp chopped parsley
2 tsp vinegar

Grill the tuna for 3 minutes on each side. Meanwhile, mix together the tomatoes, onions, chives, parsley and vinegar in a bowl. Place the tuna on four plates, spoon some salsa next to each steak, and serve immediately.

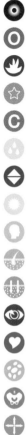

Salmon

Vitamins A, B1, B2, B3, B5, B6, B12, D, E, biotin, folic acid; calcium,
iodine, iron, magnesium, phosphorus, potassium, selenium, zinc;
omega-3 fatty acids, dimethylaminoethenol, docosahexaenoic acid,
eicosapentaenoic acid; protein; tryptophan

Containing a wealth of omega-3 fatty acids, vitamins and minerals, salmon is essential to a good diet.

Being an oily fish, salmon is an excellent source of omega-3 fatty acids in the form of eicosapentaenoic acid (EPA) and docosahexaenoic acid (DHA), which counteract many of the effects of aging and help to reduce post-exercise joint stiffness. The DHA is especially important for the brain and the nervous system, keeping the memory working well, and is believed to boost intelligence in children. By preserving brain and cell functions, the fatty acids protect against numerous diseases including cancers, stroke and dementia. They regulate the activity of white blood cells and exhibit anti-inflammatory properties.

Omega-3 fatty acids also help to control cholesterol and fat levels, thereby protecting the cardiovascular system and reducing the risk of heart disease. They aid blood flow through the arteries, prevent arrhythmia, lower blood pressure and make the blood less likely to clot. Essential fatty acids are also good for keeping the skin and hair youthful, and for combatting skin conditions, such as psoriasis and eczema.

Salmon provides plenty of low-fat protein, making it a wonderful food for regular exercisers and athletes, who need a plentiful supply of protein to help recovery time after training and to build up their muscles and stamina.

The fish contains many antioxidants, including vitamin A, which helps to keep the blood and nervous systems healthy; vitamin D, which aids calcium absorption and is good for general bone health; and selenium, a powerful antioxidant mineral, that also helps to produce antibodies and boosts immunity.

It is advisable to buy wild rather than farmed salmon in order to maximize the benefits from eating this tasty fish. Wild salmon is rich in astaxanthin, one of the most potent antioxidants ever discovered.

SALMON FISHCAKES *serves 2*

2 small salmon fillets, skinless
  and boneless
4 small potatoes, peeled and chopped
1 onion, finely chopped
2 tbsp olive oil
1 egg, beaten
1 handful parsley, chopped

Steam the salmon for 20 minutes until cooked through. Boil and lightly mash the potatoes. Sauté the onion in 1 tablespoon of oil until soft. Mix all the ingredients (except the remaining oil) and form into 8 fishcakes. Chill for 1 hour. Gently fry the fishcakes in the remaining oil until crisp on both sides. Serve.

SIZZLING SALMON

500g/1lb 2oz salmon fillets
½ tsp crushed dried chillies
¼ tsp paprika
4 tsp olive oil
salt and ground black pepper
4 tsp chopped coriander leaves, to serve

Cut the salmon into four. Place skin-side down on a griddle pan and sprinkle with the chillies, paprika and oil. Season with salt and pepper, and cook for 6–8 minutes. Sprinkle the salmon with the chopped coriander. Serve immediately.

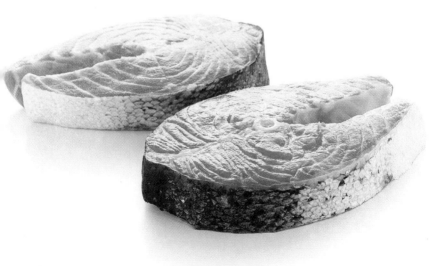

SALMON PATTIES

85g/3oz/scant ½ cup long-grain rice

1 egg

1 garlic clove

1 onion, halved

2 tsp sunflower oil, plus extra for frying

500g/1lb 2oz salmon fillets, skinned and
    chopped

1 tbsp chopped parsley

In a pan, bring 125ml/4fl oz/½ cup water to the boil. Add the rice, reduce the heat and simmer for 10 minutes. Allow to cool. In a food processor, purée the egg, garlic, onion and oil. Mix well with the rice, salmon and parsley, and form into 8 patties. Fry in batches in the oil for 4–5 minutes on each side.

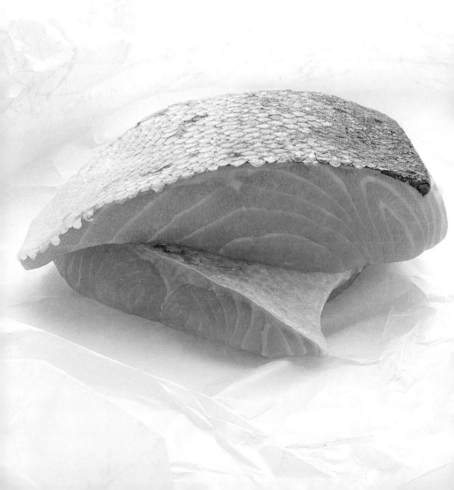

WATERCRESS SALMON STEAKS

4 salmon steaks
4 tsp extra virgin olive oil
juice of 1 lemon
1 bunch watercress, chopped
4 tbsp mayonnaise
1 tsp Tabasco sauce (optional)

Put the salmon on a grill pan. Drizzle 1 teaspoon of olive oil and lemon over each. Grill each side under medium heat for 5 minutes. Put the watercress, mayonnaise and remaining lemon juice in a blender and whizz until smooth. Season and add the Tabasco, if using. Spoon over the salmon and serve.

SALMON IN GRAPE SAUCE

2 tsp mustard
2 tsp dried thyme
2 tsp clear honey
4 salmon fillets
1 tbsp olive oil
225g/8oz seedless red grapes, halved
125ml/4fl oz/½ cup red wine

Preheat the oven to 150°C/300°F/gas mark 2. Mix together the mustard, thyme and honey and rub into the fish. Heat half the oil in a pan and brown both sides of the salmon. Transfer to an oiled baking tray and bake for 10 minutes. Heat the remaining oil in a pan and sauté the grapes for 2 minutes, add the wine, bring to the boil and reduce by half. Pour over the salmon and serve.

BAKED SALMON WITH CAPER AND TOMATO DRESSING

4 salmon fillets
2 tbsp olive oil, plus extra for greasing
1 tbsp capers, chopped
4 cherry tomatoes, chopped
1 shallot, chopped
1 tbsp lemon juice

Preheat the oven to 200°C/400°F/gas mark 6. Put each fillet on a piece of greased foil. Mix the other ingredients in a bowl and spoon over the fillets. Fold the foil to form parcels. Bake on a baking tray for 10 minutes or until cooked. Serve.

Sardine

Vitamins B3, B6, D, E; calcium, iodine, iron, phosphorus, potassium, selenium, zinc; omega-3 essential fatty acids; protein

Fresh and tinned sardines contain a host of age-defying and health-promoting fatty acids and antioxidants.

Some of the most beneficial nutrients for keeping our skin looking young and radiant are omega-3 fatty acids, and sardines are an excellent source. Research suggests that they may also help to protect the skin against sun exposure and ultra-violet radiation. However, the benefits of omega-3 fats are more than skin-deep. Several studies show that they help to make the blood less liable to clot and so reduce the risk of heart disease. They also keep the eyes healthy and boost brain function.

Packed with protein, iron and zinc, sardines are exceptionally rich in calcium. Being one of the few non-dairy sources of easily absorbable calcium makes them a first-rate food for athletes. Sardines are also an excellent source of vitamin D, which is vital for healthy bones because it increases the body's ability to absorb calcium. In addition, sardines are high in selenium, a powerful antioxidant that helps to prevent wrinkles and heart disease. Selenium is anti-carcinogenic and neutralizes toxic metals in the body.

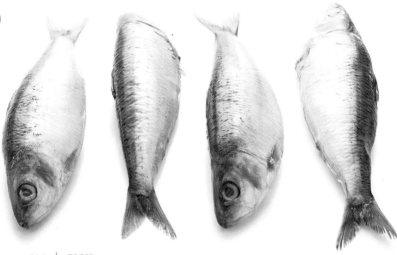

GRILLED SARDINES WITH SALSA VERDE

2 large onions, chopped
2 garlic cloves, peeled
2 large green peppers, deseeded and
  chopped
125ml/4fl oz/½ cup extra virgin olive oil
50g/2oz tinned anchovies, drained
2 small green chillies, deseeded
juice and grated zest of 2 lemons
2 tbsp capers
2 large handfuls chopped basil
1 large handful chopped parsley
12 fresh sardines

In a saucepan, gently sauté the onion, garlic and peppers with half the oil. Put in a food processor with the anchovies, chillies, lemon juice and zest, capers and herbs and whizz into a chunky purée. Grill the sardines on foil under a hot grill for 5–7 minutes on each side. Place on a serving plate, drizzle over the salsa and serve.

JAPANESE SARDINES

450g/1lb sardines, gutted, washed
  and dried
125ml/4fl oz/½ cup soy sauce
4 tbsp white wine vinegar
juice and zest of 1 lime
1 lemon grass stalk, chopped
2.5cm/1in piece root ginger, peeled
  and chopped
2 garlic cloves, crushed
1 tsp chilli powder

Arrange the sardines in a shallow dish. Mix together the remaining ingredients in a bowl and pour over the sardines. Cover and refrigerate for 3 hours. Discard the marinade and grill the sardines, turning once, for 5 minutes on each side or until the flesh flakes.

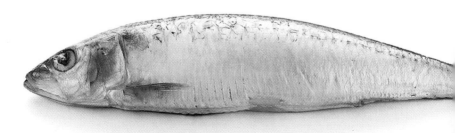

Prawn

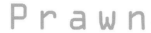

VITAMINS B3, B12; CALCIUM, IODINE, MAGNESIUM, PHOSPHORUS, POTASSIUM, SELENIUM, SODIUM, ZINC; PROTEIN

The world's most popular and versatile crustaceans, immunity-boosting prawns work well in sandwiches, salads, stir-fries and seafood stews.

Prawns are a great source of protein, which is necessary for building healthy bones and muscles as well as for boosting energy. They are rich in vitamin B3, which is crucial for preserving the memory, and vitamin B12, which promotes brain function and prevents fatigue.

Prawns contain high levels of immune-essential minerals, including zinc, which we need to produce the enzymes that keep cancer at bay, and to help to develop other disease-fighting cells. This mineral also boosts fertility. The shellfish contain selenium, a potent antioxidant mineral that helps in the production of antibodies and improves the efficiency of white blood cells at recognizing unwanted invaders, as well as fighting off wrinkles. In addition, prawns supply iodine, which is vital for the proper functioning of the thyroid gland, and calcium and phosphorus for strong bones. Phosphorus also regulates red blood cell metabolism.

Prawns are a particularly good food for athletes, and sportsmen and -women. They are loaded with vital minerals, including potassium, magnesium and sodium, that all help to balance the body's water levels and to restore the electrolyte balance after a session of exercise or a sport's match. As prawns are higher in sodium content than most foods (although not in harmful levels), they can also help to prevent the mineral imbalance that can result from drinking too much water during an energetic workout.

PRAWNS WITH PEPPER SAUCE

4 red peppers, deseeded and chopped

1 tomato, chopped

2 garlic cloves, crushed

2 tbsp chopped parsley

1 tbsp white wine vinegar

800g/1lb 12oz cooked prawns

1 iceberg lettuce

Place the peppers on a baking tray and bake for 10 minutes or until soft. Mix together in a bowl with the tomato, garlic, parsley and vinegar. Shred the lettuce and divide among four bowls. Peel the prawns and place a few in each bowl, before topping with the pepper mixture.

PRAWN PÂTÉ

450g/1lb cooked, peeled prawns

40g/1½ oz butter

3 tbsp cream cheese

1 tbsp sour cream

2 drops Tabasco sauce

½ tsp ground nutmeg

1 garlic clove, crushed

1 tbsp lemon juice

salt and ground black pepper

Put the prawns (reserving one) in a blender with all the other ingredients. Whizz until smooth. Place the pâté in a serving dish and garnish with the whole prawn.

PRAWNS AND BULGUR WHEAT

225g/8oz/1¼ cups bulgur wheat

500ml/17fl oz/2 cups hot
   vegetable stock

1 red onion, finely diced

400g/14oz cooked,
   peeled prawns

2 handfuls basil,
   chopped

Place the bulgur wheat in a pan, pour over the stock and leave to stand for 30 minutes. Stir in the raw onion, prawns and basil, and serve.

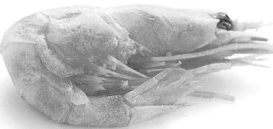

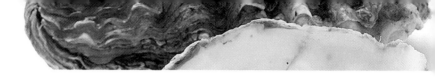

Oyster

Vitamins A, B3, B12, C, D, E; calcium, copper, iodine, iron, magnesium, potassium, selenium, zinc; omega-3 fatty acids; protein

Oysters are a type of shellfish that is not only a renowned aphrodisiac but is also full of health-promoting vitamins, minerals and other nutrients.

A versatile food, oysters can be cooked in many ways, including roasting, baking, grilling, frying, stewing, boiling and steaming. They are also available tinned, smoked and pickled. However, they are traditionally eaten raw with a pinch of salt or a dash of lemon juice.

The nutritional value of oysters and their flavour and texture can vary according to the type of water in which they grow, as they are affected by factors such as salinity levels and mineral content.

A great source of energy for athletes, oysters are an excellent form of low-fat protein. They are loaded with vitamin E, which is also good for the skin and for preventing heart disease, as well as conditions such as arthritis. The shellfish are a very rich, low-fat source of omega-3 fatty acids, which are vital for heart health and make us feel happier and livelier by supporting the brain's healthy functioning.

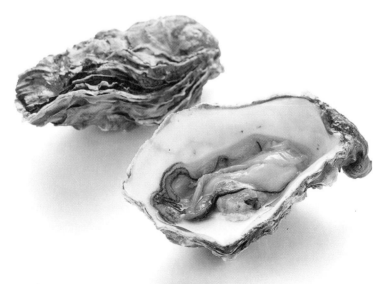

Oysters are also full of B-vitamins, essential to mind and mood, including B12, which helps to fight fatigue. They are an excellent source of the mineral iodine, vital for the proper functioning of the thyroid gland, which, if under-active, can lead to debilitating bouts of exhaustion.

The shellfish also contain vitamin D, which is needed for healthy bones and teeth, as well as potassium and iron, which combat anaemia. In Chinese medicine, the shellfish supplement the liver and kidneys, and treat insomnia, restlessness and agitation.

Packed with nutrients, oysters act as a general health tonic as well as enhancing sexual well-being. They have a well-documented affinity with the reproductive system. Research also indicates that certain sterols are present in oysters, from which the sex hormones are derived. They are used regularly by Chinese women to increase oestrogen in the body, and are useful for infertility and for treating menopausal disorders.

Oysters are a rich natural source of nutrients, including zinc – just six raw oysters provide excellent amounts of this important nutrient. Zinc is essential for the production of sperm, and restores libido to people who don't enjoy sex any more. When the body is short of vital nutrients, sex is low on the list of functions it needs to maintain. Zinc also helps to boost immunity, maintain youthful skin and prevent hair loss.

OYSTERS AU PARMESAN

125g/4½oz/1 cup fresh breadcrumbs
15g/½oz butter, plus extra for greasing
36 fresh oysters, shelled
1 handful chopped parsley
125g /4½oz/1 cup freshly grated
  Parmesan cheese
125ml/4fl oz/½ cup white wine
salt and cayenne pepper

Preheat the oven to 180°C/350°F/ gas mark 4. In a pan, brown the breadcrumbs in the butter, reserving 1 tablespoon of the crumbs. Grease a shallow baking dish, then dust with the fried breadcrumbs. Season the oysters with salt and cayenne pepper and place them on top of the breadcrumbs. Scatter the parsley and Parmesan on top, followed by the reserved breadcrumbs. Pour the wine over the entire dish. Bake in the oven for 15 minutes. Serve hot.

OYSTER BISQUE

24 fresh oysters, shelled
455ml/16fl oz/scant 2 cups vegetable stock
900ml/32fl oz/4 cups milk
225ml/8fl oz/1 cup single cream
1 tbsp potato flour
1 tbsp butter
salt and white pepper

In a saucepan, simmer the oysters in the stock for about 30 minutes. Strain, then add the milk and cream and season to taste. Simmer gently for 2 minutes. Mix the potato flour with the butter, add to the saucepan and stir to thicken. Serve.

GREEN OYSTERS

24 fresh oysters
450g/1lb spinach, chopped
115g/4oz parsley, chopped
4 tbsp white wine

Preheat the oven to 220°C/425°F/gas mark 7. Open the oysters, remove from the shells and wash, discarding any already open. Place on half shells in a baking dish. Mix together the spinach, parsley and white wine. Spread over the oysters and bake for 6–7 minutes, until cooked through, and serve.

ROASTED OYSTERS

16 fresh oysters
1 tbsp sesame oil
1 tbsp white wine vinegar
1 tbsp lemon juice
1cm/½ in piece root ginger, peeled
   and grated
1 tsp salt

Preheat the oven to 200°C/400°F/gas mark 6. Place the oysters deep-shell down on a roasting tray and roast for 5 minutes until they open. Whisk the sesame oil, white wine vinegar, lemon juice, ginger and salt in a bowl. Flip off the top shells, and add a drizzle of dressing to each oyster. Serve the oysters in their shells as a starter.

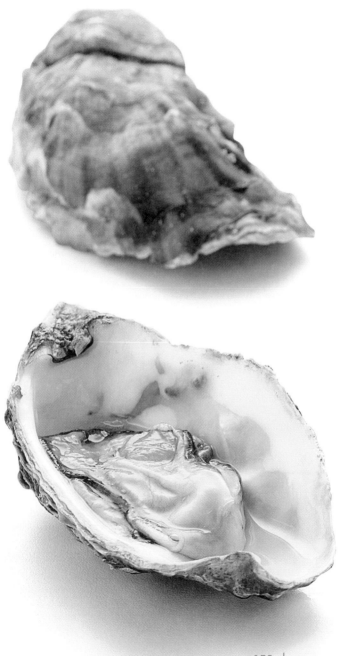

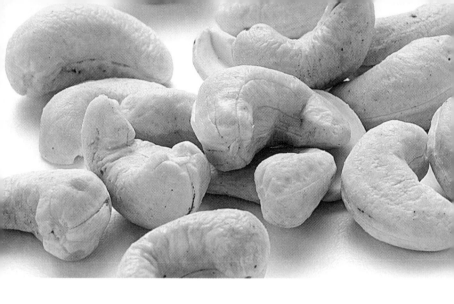

LITTLE POWERHOUSES
OF GOODNESS, NUTS AND
SEEDS ARE BRIMMING
WITH ENERGY, MAKING
THEM FANTASTIC SNACKS
AT ANY TIME

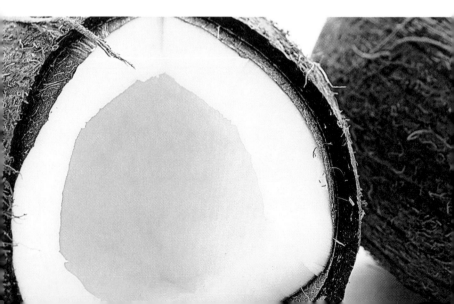

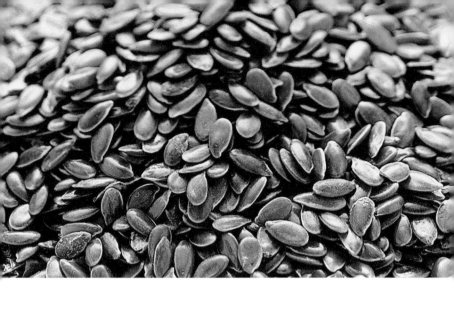

05 | **wonder**
NUTS, SEEDS
& OIL'S

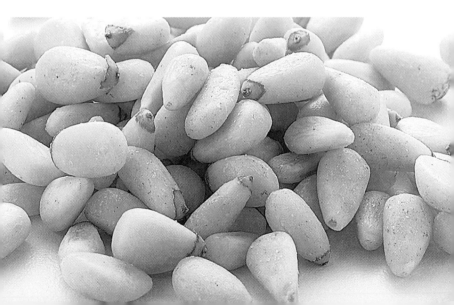

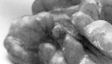
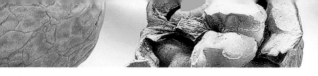

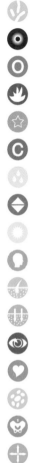

Walnut

VITAMINS B1, B2, B3, B5, B6, E, BIOTIN, FOLIC ACID; CALCIUM, COPPER, IODINE, IRON, MAGNESIUM, MANGANESE, PHOSPHORUS, POTASSIUM, SELENIUM, ZINC; OMEGA-3, -6 AND -9 FATTY ACIDS; GLUTATHIONE; ARGININE; ELLAGIC ACID; PROTEIN; TRYPTOPHAN; FIBRE

Walnuts are a wonderful snack food, providing many nutrients as well as a healthy oil. With their two-lobed appearance resembling a brain, it's no surprise that walnuts aid cognitive function and sharpen the memory.

One of the richest sources of antioxidants, walnuts protect the heart in numerous ways, preventing arrhythmia as well as lowering cholesterol and protecting the arteries. Walnuts contain glutathione, an important antioxidant that aids the development of lymphocyte cells and thereby boosts immunity.

Walnuts and walnut oil contain protein, vitamins B6 and E, potassium, magnesium, copper and zinc, all of which help to keep us youthful. Vitamin B6 helps to prevent memory loss and protect the heart, while vitamin E maintains healthy skin and hair. Both potassium and magnesium are good for the heart, and copper helps to prevent varicose veins. Zinc has a miraculous ability to rejuvenate the thymus gland and to boost immunity.

One of walnut's most valuable effects is in fighting inflammation. This means a lot more than just relieving sore skin and painful joints, especially as you grow older. Inflammation plays a role in many of the most debilitating conditions of age. It hardens the arteries, causing high blood pressure, strokes and heart disease. It speeds up thinning of the bones, leading to osteoporosis. The damage caused by chronic inflammation has been linked with the development of cancers. And it is implicated in degenerative diseases of both brain and body. Eating just half a dozen

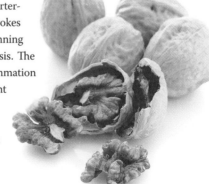

walnuts a day is enough to reduce your risk. Furthermore, scientists have found that eating walnuts at the end of a rich meal can counter the potentially harmful effects of the fat you've eaten by reducing inflammation and keeping the arteries clear.

Walnuts may reduce the risk of developing diabetes, but if you already have it, they provide the right balance of fats in your diet. They are not only a good source of heart-healthy monounsaturated fats but also contain alpha-linolenic acid, an omega-3 essential fatty acid, which makes them unique among nuts. Omega-3 fats provide cardiovascular protection and aid brain function and positive mood; they're also anti-inflammatory and so are useful in the treatment of asthma, rheumatoid arthritis and skin disorders, such as eczema and psoriasis. In addition, walnuts contain the amino acid arginine, which helps to keep blood vessels flexible, and ellagic acid, an antioxidant that research has shown to have powerful anti-cancer properties.

WALNUT PASTA SALAD

4 tbsp chopped walnuts,
350g /12oz/3¾ cups wholemeal pasta
   spirals, cooked
3 large tomatoes, cut into wedges
1 handful rocket
2 tbsp chopped basil
1 garlic clove, crushed
4 tbsp walnut oil
2 tbsp balsamic vinegar

In a large bowl, combine all the ingredients except the garlic, oil and vinegar. Whisk these remaining ingredients together, then drizzle over the salad. Serve immediately.

WALNUT AND BANANA WHIRL

2 bananas, chopped
250ml/9fl oz/1 cup plain bio-yogurt
60g/2¼oz/½ cup chopped walnuts
2 tbsp clear honey

Place the bananas in a blender. Add the yogurt, half the walnuts and the honey. Blend, on a low speed at first, until smooth. Serve immediately, topped with the remaining walnuts.

WALNUT, APPLE AND CELERY STUFFING

1 large onion, chopped
2 celery stalks, trimmed and chopped
85g/3oz butter
2 cooking apples, peeled, cored and chopped
350g/12oz fresh breadcrumbs
225g/8oz/2 cups chopped walnuts
½ tsp dried thyme
1 large egg, beaten
125ml/4fl oz/½ cup milk

Preheat the oven to 180°C/350°F/gas mark 4. Fry the onion and celery in the butter in a pan. Mix the apples, breadcrumbs, walnuts and thyme in a bowl; stir in the vegetables, egg and milk. Spoon into a baking dish. Bake for 30 minutes, then serve.

SPICY WALNUTS

1 tbsp curry paste
1 tsp mango juice
1 tsp ground cumin
115g/4oz/1 cup walnuts

Preheat the oven to 180°C/350°F/gas mark 4. Mix together the curry paste, mango juice and cumin into a smooth paste. Coat the walnuts and place on an oiled baking tray and cook for 5–10 minutes until crisp. Serve as a snack.

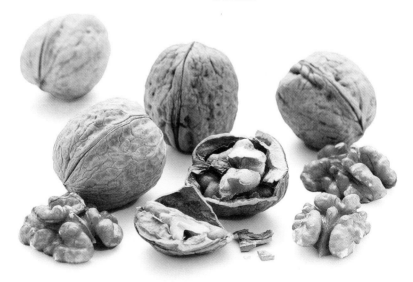

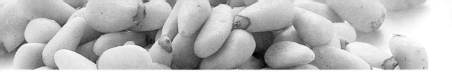

Pine nut

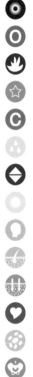

Vitamins B1, B2, B3, E; copper, iron, magnesium, manganese, zinc; pinoleic acid; omega-6 essential fatty acids; protein

Full of protein and minerals, these aromatic kernels can aid the prevention of disease. They are perfect with pasta, in stir-fries or salads, or as an energy-boosting snack.

The small edible seeds of the pine tree, pine nuts are lower in fat content than most other nuts, which means they're a brilliant choice for weight-conscious athletes who need to get plenty of muscle-building protein and joint-friendly essential fats in their diet without overloading on calories.

As well as being rich in the immunity-boosting antioxidant zinc, pine nuts contain high levels of anti-inflammatory polyunsaturated fats, which help to maintain low cholesterol and promote a healthy heart. They are high in immunity-boosting vitamin E, which helps to protect against damage caused by pollution and other toxins, and is needed by the immune system's antibodies to fight disease. In addition, pine nuts are a good source of magnesium, which helps to calm allergic reactions.

Pine nuts are also nature's only source of pinoleic acid, which stimulates the secretion of a hormone in the gut that sends messages to the brain indicating that you are full. The brain then switches off the appetite. Pinoleic acid also slows the rate at which food leaves the stomach, leaving you feeling fuller for longer.

RED PEPPER BRUSCHETTA

4 red peppers, deseeded and sliced
1 garlic clove, crushed
1 tbsp balsamic vinegar
5 tbsp olive oil
1 wholemeal loaf, thickly sliced
200g/7oz goats' cheese, sliced
55g/2oz/⅓ cup pine nuts, toasted

Grill the peppers until soft, then place in a bowl and toss with the garlic, vinegar and 4 tbsp of the oil. Drizzle the remaining oil over the bread, and place in a hot oven to bake until golden on each side, turning once. Top each slice with goats' cheese, peppers and pine nuts.

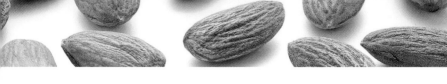

Almond

Vitamins B1, B2, B3, B5, B6, E, biotin, folic acid; calcium, copper, iodine, iron, magnesium, manganese, phosphorus, potassium, selenium, zinc; monounsaturated fats, omega-6 essential fatty acids, omega-9 fatty acids; laetrile; plant sterols; protein; fibre

These strongly flavoured nuts contain healthy oils and other vitality-enhancing nutrients. Nibbling on almonds provides nutrients and energy for people who work out, with less risk of piling on unwanted kilos/pounds.

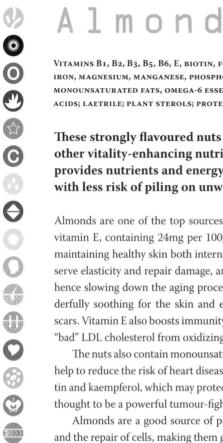

Almonds are one of the top sources of cancer-preventing antioxidant vitamin E, containing 24mg per 100g. This plays an important role in maintaining healthy skin both internally and externally, helping to preserve elasticity and repair damage, and protect cells from free radicals, hence slowing down the aging process. Almond oil, especially, is wonderfully soothing for the skin and effective in healing post-operative scars. Vitamin E also boosts immunity and protects the heart by keeping "bad" LDL cholesterol from oxidizing and sticking to artery walls.

The nuts also contain monounsaturated fats and plant sterols, which help to reduce the risk of heart disease, and the phytochemicals quercetin and kaempferol, which may protect against cancer, as well as laetrile, thought to be a powerful tumour-fighting compound.

Almonds are a good source of protein, needed for healthy growth and the repair of cells, making them great for vegetarians. The nuts also contain more fibre than any other nut, which helps almonds to promote healthy digestion through the efficient elimination of waste matter. They are full of calcium, which aids muscle function and helps to keep bones strong and to stave off osteoporosis. Almonds also provide zinc, magnesium and potassium. While zinc strengthens immunity and improves wound healing, magnesium increases energy and potassium reduces blood pressure, protecting against heart disease.

Almonds are a useful food for dieters. They may seem an odd weight-loss choice because they contain quite a lot of fat, but when scientists put two groups of people on low-calorie diets, one of which included almonds, the almond-eating group lost 50 per cent more weight and fat than the others. Almonds are rich in monounsaturated fat, which helps you feel fuller for longer, and their high fibre content helps to keep blood-sugar levels steady and prevent hunger pangs. A dozen almonds contain just 90 calories along with a burst of protein and nutrients that combine to increase energy levels, so they are a great snack food for athletes, and sportsmen and -women.

ALMOND AND RAISIN MILK

225g/8oz/2 cups whole almonds
 (not roasted or salted)
1 handful dried raisins
455ml/16fl oz/scant 2 cups water

Cover the almonds with water and soak for 24 hours; drain and rinse. Soak the raisins in water for 2 hours, then drain. Put the almonds, raisins and the water in a food processor. Blend, then strain through a fine sieve and drink. Keeps in the fridge for up to 4 days.

ALMOND BANANA SMOOTHIE

150g/5½oz/1 cup blanched almonds
2 small bananas
a pinch of cinnamon
2 tsp vanilla extract
2 tsp clear honey

Place the almonds, bananas and 500ml/17fl oz/2 cups water in a blender and whizz until smooth. Add the vanilla extract, honey and cinnamon and whizz again. Serve.

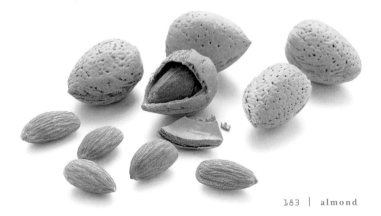

ALMOND MACAROONS

2 large egg whites
175g/6oz/1¾ cups ground almonds
85g/3oz/⅓ cup caster sugar
1 tsp almond extract
a pinch of salt

Preheat the oven to 180°C/350°F/gas mark 4. In a bowl, whisk the egg whites to form firm peaks. Fold in the almonds and sugar, then the almond extract and salt. Roll out and cut into 20 rounds. Place on a greased baking tray and bake for 20 minutes until golden. Cool on a wire rack.

RASPBERRY ALMOND BAKE

450g/1lb raspberry jam
1 egg, beaten
5 tbsp brown rice syrup
100g/3½oz/1 cup ground almonds
4 tbsp sunflower oil
5 tbsp rice milk
½ tsp natural vanilla extract
4 drops almond extract

Preheat the oven to 190°C/375°F/gas mark 5. Spread the jam over the base of an ovenproof dish. Put the remaining ingredients in a bowl, mix well and spoon the mixture evenly over the jam. Bake for 40–45 minutes until golden and firm to the touch.

*TRADITIONAL ALMOND MILK
to nourish the skin

50g/1¾ oz/½ cup ground almonds
2 tbsp clear honey
500ml/17fl oz/2 cups still mineral water

In a bowl, combine the almonds, honey and water. Stir well, until the honey has dissolved. Leave for 2 hours. Filter, and pour into a bottle with a lid. Apply generously to the face and neck with cotton wool, and leave on for 20 minutes. Use in the morning and evening. Keeps for up to 3 days in the fridge.

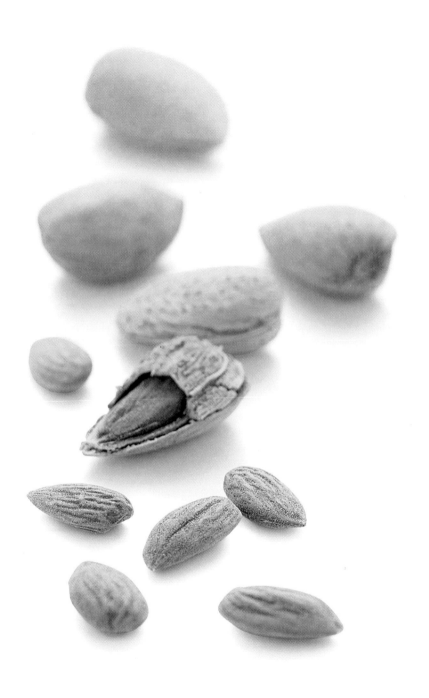

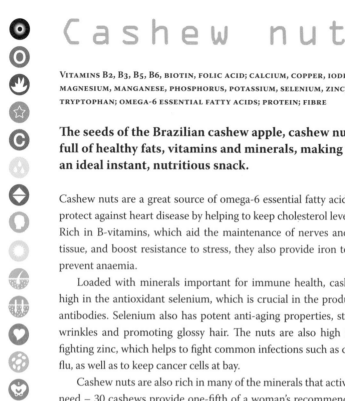

Cashew nut

Vitamins B2, B3, B5, B6, biotin, folic acid; calcium, copper, iodine, iron, magnesium, manganese, phosphorus, potassium, selenium, zinc; tryptophan; omega-6 essential fatty acids; protein; fibre

The seeds of the Brazilian cashew apple, cashew nuts are full of healthy fats, vitamins and minerals, making them an ideal instant, nutritious snack.

Cashew nuts are a great source of omega-6 essential fatty acids, which protect against heart disease by helping to keep cholesterol levels down. Rich in B-vitamins, which aid the maintenance of nerves and muscle tissue, and boost resistance to stress, they also provide iron to help to prevent anaemia.

Loaded with minerals important for immune health, cashews are high in the antioxidant selenium, which is crucial in the production of antibodies. Selenium also has potent anti-aging properties, staving off wrinkles and promoting glossy hair. The nuts are also high in virus-fighting zinc, which helps to fight common infections such as colds and flu, as well as to keep cancer cells at bay.

Cashew nuts are also rich in many of the minerals that active people need – 30 cashews provide one-fifth of a woman's recommended daily iron intake, while 20 nuts provide more than one-tenth of a man's daily zinc requirement. The phosphorus in the nuts works with the calcium to form and maintain strong bones, while the copper has healing properties, and may help to rid the body of infections.

Cashews are packed with the minerals essential to fitness: magnesium keeps bones strong while combating muscle fatigue and soreness. They also aid the function of the heart and enable the metabolism of calcium, which prevents osteoporosis. In addition, the copper in cashews not only increases energy and protects joints from injury but also helps the body to utilize iron.

There is no handier snack than a packet of nuts after you've worked up an appetite exercising. The body is still burning calories faster than usual up to an hour or so after a workout, so make the most of this and enjoy some healthy cashews rather than an empty-calorie snack.

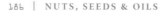

SUMMER BERRIES WITH CASHEW CREAM

150g/5½oz/1 cup cashew nuts

1 tsp ground nutmeg

2 tbsp clear honey

200g/7oz/1¼ cups raspberries

200g/7oz/1⅓ cups strawberries,
   hulled and halved

Blend the nuts and 100ml/3½fl oz/⅓ cup water in a food processor until smooth, then add the nutmeg and honey and whizz again until thoroughly blended. Divide the berries into four bowls, top with the cashew cream and serve.

CHICKEN WITH CASHEWS

1 tbsp groundnut oil

2 bird's eye chillies, deseeded and chopped

5cm/2in piece root ginger, finely chopped

450g/1lb skinless chicken breasts, cubed

2 spring onions, trimmed and chopped

2 tsp vinegar

2 tsp sesame oil

2 heaped tbsp cashew nuts

rice, to serve

Heat the groundnut oil and briefly stir-fry the chillies and ginger. Add the chicken and stir-fry for 2–3 minutes. Add the spring onions, vinegar and sesame oil and fry for 5 minutes, until the chicken is cooked. Transfer to a bowl. Stir-fry the cashews for 1 minute and sprinkle over the chicken. Serve with rice.

CASHEW NUT DIP

115g/4oz/¾ cup cashew nuts

1 tbsp crunchy peanut butter

3 garlic cloves, crushed

3 tbsp olive oil

juice of 1 lemon

100g/3½oz/⅓ cup tahini

a pinch of paprika

pitta bread, to serve

Blend all the ingredients in a food processor until smooth. Serve with pitta bread.

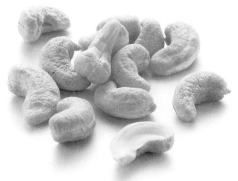

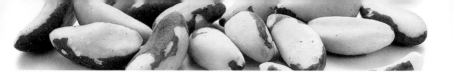

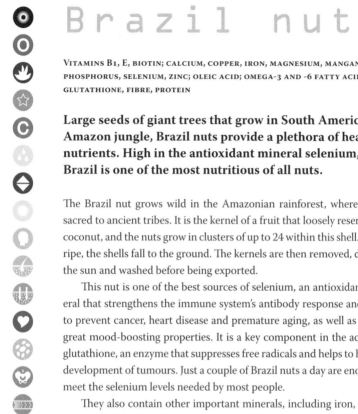

Brazil nut

Vitamins B1, E, biotin; calcium, copper, iron, magnesium, manganese, phosphorus, selenium, zinc; oleic acid; omega-3 and -6 fatty acids; glutathione, fibre, protein

Large seeds of giant trees that grow in South America's Amazon jungle, Brazil nuts provide a plethora of healing nutrients. High in the antioxidant mineral selenium, the Brazil is one of the most nutritious of all nuts.

The Brazil nut grows wild in the Amazonian rainforest, where it was sacred to ancient tribes. It is the kernel of a fruit that loosely resembles a coconut, and the nuts grow in clusters of up to 24 within this shell. When ripe, the shells fall to the ground. The kernels are then removed, dried in the sun and washed before being exported.

This nut is one of the best sources of selenium, an antioxidant mineral that strengthens the immune system's antibody response and helps to prevent cancer, heart disease and premature aging, as well as having great mood-boosting properties. It is a key component in the action of glutathione, an enzyme that suppresses free radicals and helps to halt the development of tumours. Just a couple of Brazil nuts a day are enough to meet the selenium levels needed by most people.

They also contain other important minerals, including iron, crucial for healthy blood, and magnesium, essential to the nervous system and important for the formation of protein, and for boosting energy.

Brazil nuts are packed with vitamin E, which works with selenium to provide a super-boost to the immune system, and also contain vitamin B1, which is essential to the nervous system.

Brazil nuts are about 70 per cent fat. Half of this is oleic acid, the building block for the omega-9 fatty acids that are excellent for the skin and have anti-inflammatory properties. The rest is made up of omega-6 and omega-3 essential fatty acids, which promote healthy skin, glossy hair and a good memory, ease inflammation and enhance digestion.

Rich in protein, a handful of Brazil nuts eaten raw makes a satisfying snack. They can be processed into nut milk or butter, and can be used in stir-fries and salads to add a crunchy protein kick.

GREEN BEAN AND BRAZIL NUT STIR-FRY

2 tbsp sesame oil
1 onion, chopped
1 tbsp grated fresh ginger
2 garlic cloves, crushed
200g/7oz asparagus spears
200g/7oz green beans
100g/3½oz/¾ cup Brazil nuts, sliced
2 tbsp soy sauce

Heat the sesame oil in a wok over a high heat until it is sizzling hot, then add the onion, ginger and garlic. Stir-fry for 2 minutes, then add the asparagus spears, green beans and Brazil nuts. Continue to stir-fry for a further 5 minutes, then add the soy sauce. Reduce the heat and cook slowly until the asparagus and beans are tender – this should take 8–10 minutes. Serve immediately on a bed of brown rice.

BRAZIL NUT BRITTLE

440g/15½oz/2 cups granulated sugar
¼ tsp bicarbonate of soda
190g/6¾oz/1½ cups ground Brazil nuts
175g/6oz milk chocolate, melted

In a heavy frying pan, melt the sugar over a low heat, stirring. Add the soda and 125g/4½oz/1 cup of the nuts, and mix. Roll out on a greased baking sheet until about 5mm/¼in thick. When cold, cover with the melted chocolate and sprinkle with the remaining nuts. Once set, break into pieces.

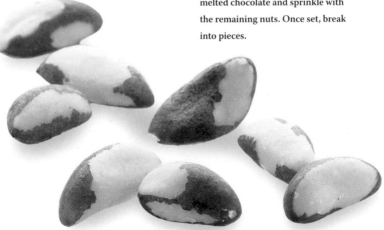

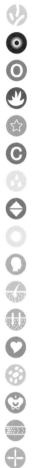

Coconut and coconut oil

VITAMINS B1, B2, B3, B5, B6, C, E, FOLIC ACID; CALCIUM, COPPER, IODINE, IRON, MAGNESIUM, MANGANESE, PHOSPHORUS, POTASSIUM, SELENIUM, ZINC; FIBRE; PROTEIN; CARBOHYDRATE; MEDIUM CHAIN FATTY ACIDS

Traditionally the staple food on many tropical islands, this health-giving nut has potent healing properties.

Although coconut is high in saturated fats, they're a different type to those found in meat and dairy and don't pose the same health risks. Known as medium chain fatty acids (MCFAs), they are soluble and easily digested and metabolized by the body, and are used as an energy source rather than being stored as fat. MCFAs have been shown to assist the absorption of calcium, magnesium and some amino acids, as well as supporting the healthy function of the thyroid. They also stimulate metabolism, benefit the heart and promote weight loss.

Rich in vitamins, coconut oil's vitamin E keeps the skin's connective tissues strong and supple, which helps to prevent wrinkles.

The coconut water – the liquid inside young coconuts – is known to be one of the most balanced electrolyte sources in nature, making a wonderful rehydration drink following intense exercise or when fluids and electrolytes have been lost through diarrhoea or fever.

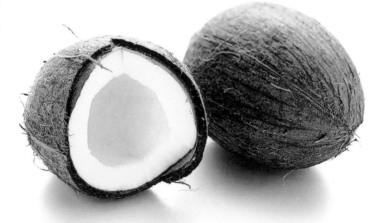

✳ COCONUT BODY OIL *to moisturize the skin*

80ml/2½fl oz/⅓ cup coconut oil in a tub
15 drops of your favourite essential oil

Remove the lid from the coconut oil and place the tub in a large pan with water; heat gently, until the oil liquefies. Add your favourite essential oil and stir well. Replace the lid and put the tub in the fridge for 15 minutes. Apply generously all over your body (but not to your face). Beware that the oil could stain your clothes, so avoid dressing until the oil has soaked well into the skin.

NON-ALCOHOLIC PIÑA COLADA

500ml/17fl oz/2 cups pineapple juice
200ml/7fl oz/¾ cup coconut water
200g/7oz tinned pineapple in fruit juice
55g/2oz creamed coconut

Put all the ingredients in a blender and whizz until smooth. Pour into a glass pitcher and stir well before serving with ice.

COCONUT RICE

225g/8oz/1 cup brown rice
1 onion, chopped
1 tbsp ground coriander
1 tbsp ground cumin
2 tbsp coconut oil
2 beef tomatoes, chopped
3 tbsp desiccated coconut

Place the rice and 500ml/17fl oz/ 2 cups water in a pan and bring to the boil. Reduce the heat and simmer for 45 minutes. In another pan, fry the onion and spices in the oil for 3 minutes. Add the tomatoes and coconut, and simmer for 10 minutes. Mix well with the rice. Serve as a side dish.

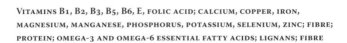

Flaxseed

VITAMINS B1, B2, B3, B5, B6, E, FOLIC ACID; CALCIUM, COPPER, IRON, MAGNESIUM, MANGANESE, PHOSPHORUS, POTASSIUM, SELENIUM, ZINC; FIBRE; PROTEIN; OMEGA-3 AND OMEGA-6 ESSENTIAL FATTY ACIDS; LIGNANS; FIBRE

With abundant and balanced levels of essential fatty acids, flaxseed is acclaimed in history for its ability to prevent and combat many conditions. This tiny wonderfood, also known as linseed, can lift depression, aid concentration, increase energy levels and smooth hormonal changes.

Today, the amazing health-giving virtues of flaxseed are recognized throughout the world. Whatever your age or sex, flaxseed could make you feel happier and help you to think more clearly. This superseed contains nutrients that are vital to brain functioning but often lacking in people's everyday diets.

Flaxseed is one of the richest sources of alpha-linolenic acid (ALA), an omega-3 essential fatty acid renowned for its benefits to both mind and body. One of the ways in which omega-3s help to keep the brain and nervous system working smoothly is by allowing cells to function and communicate with each other properly. This can prevent many disorders that we think of as psychological. It also increases mental alertness and boosts memory. Our ability to use omega-3s is reduced by saturated and hydrogenated fats, which compete for the same receptors in our bodies. So cut down on these fats and eat foods rich in vitamins B3, B6 and C, plus zinc and magnesium, which help the body to absorb ALA.

High in omega-6 essential fatty acids (EFAs) in addition to omega-3s, flaxseeds are involved in systematic energy production, oxygen transfer and transportation of fats, and may therefore help to maintain the body's tissue cells, reproductive organs, glands, muscles and eyes. Flaxseed is thus traditionally used to treat everything from malnutrition and skin diseases to arthritis, PMS and fertility problems. For women aged over 35, it can also alleviate stressful peri-menopausal symptoms, such as hot flushes, insomnia and mood swings, as it is rich in compounds called lignans, which the body converts into substances that smooth out fluctuating hormone levels. Lignans are special compounds that are converted by friendly bacteria in the gut into phytoestrogens called enterolactone and enterodiol. These health-giving compounds have also been found to offer protection against breast cancer. (However, flaxseed oil, while rich in omega-3s, does not contain lignans and loses much of its value if used in cooking.)

Essential fatty acids are also needed to make prostaglandins, hormone-like substances responsible for stamina, circulation and metabolism. These are anti-inflammatory, and may benefit conditions such as asthma and arthritis. They also promote heart health by reducing cholesterol, blood pressure and plaque formation in the artery walls. Not only this, prostaglandins encourage weight loss by removing excess fluid from tissues and boosting metabolism, thereby helping to burn calories.

Flaxseed is expectorant and dissolving by nature and may help to treat conditions such as coughs and bronchitis, as well as other respiratory ailments. The seeds also have a mild purgative action and can be capable of tonifying the bowel, easing constipation.

Another great feature of flaxseed is mucilage, a type of soluble fibre that lowers cholesterol, stabilizes blood-sugar levels and alleviates constipation. Flaxseed's laxative effect is gentle, helping to keep intestinal contents moving smoothly along.

The benefits of flaxseed do not stop there. Its Vitamin E content helps to keep the skin looking youthful and the hair glossy. Flaxseed also contains antiviral, anti-bacterial and anti-fungal properties. Its zinc and selenium, two powerful antioxidant minerals, boost the immune system to protect against infections, while its iron and copper help in the production of haemoglobin, needed to keep red blood cells healthy. Copper also aids wound healing and the formation of collagen in the skin. In addition, the seeds provide calcium and magnesium, which together support strong, healthy bones, while magnesium also helps to ward off muscle cramps and release energy.

As flaxseeds and their oils are easily oxidized, which causes them to go rancid, keep them in dark bottles or tubs with sealed lids, and store them in the fridge for no longer than a year.

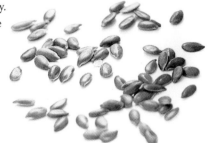

TROPICAL FLAX SHAKE

1 tbsp flaxseeds
600ml/21fl oz/2⅓ cups pineapple juice
200ml/7fl oz/¾ cup apple juice
2 kiwi fruit, peeled and chopped
2 passion fruit, halved

Grind the flaxseeds in a coffee grinder and put them in a blender along with the fruit juices and kiwi fruit. Scoop out the seeds from the passion fruit and add them to the juice mixture. Blend well and drink immediately.

FLAXSEED MUFFINS *makes 12*

115g/4oz/½ cup golden flaxseeds, ground
175g/6oz/1¼ cups wholemeal flour
1 tbsp baking powder
2 tsp ground allspice
200g/7oz/1 cup brown sugar
1 egg, beaten
250ml/9fl oz/1 cup milk

Preheat the oven to 180°C/350°F/gas mark 4. Mix the dry ingredients in a bowl. Add the egg and milk and stir together. Spoon into 12 muffin cases in a muffin tin and bake for 25 minutes. Turn out on a wire rack to cool.

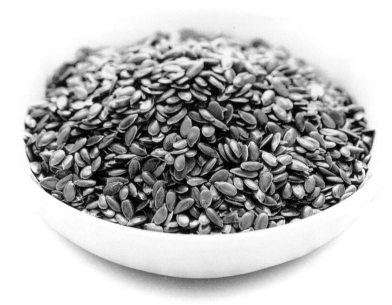

*FLAXSEED FACE MASK *to smoothe wrinkles*

2 tsp flaxseeds
1 drop neroli oil

Put the flaxseeds in a small bowl and cover with water. Leave to stand until the seeds swell and the water turns to gel, then add the neroli oil. Using your fingers, spread the gel over your face and neck. Allow to dry, then rinse off with cool or tepid water. Pat your face dry.

BREAKFAST BOOST

4 tbsp flaxseeds
2 bananas, sliced
½ small Cantaloupe melon, peeled, deseeded and chopped
4 tsp pumpkin seeds
2 tsp sesame seeds
8 tbsp/½ cup plain bio-yogurt
115g/4oz/¾ cup strawberries, hulled and chopped

Place the ingredients, except for the strawberries, in a bowl and mix together well. Serve topped with the strawberries.

PEANUT FLAX BARS

100g/3½oz/heaped ⅓ cup flaxseeds
150g/5½oz puffed rice cereal
5 tbsp crunchy peanut butter
5 tbsp brown rice syrup

Grind the flaxseeds in a nut grinder and put them in a large bowl. Add the puffed cereal, peanut butter and rice syrup, and mix well using your hands. Press the mixture very firmly into a non-stick baking tray and leave to stand for several hours before cutting into bars.

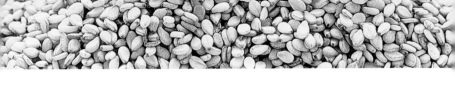

Sesame seed and oil

VITAMINS B1, B2, B3, B5, B6, E, BETA-CAROTENE; CALCIUM, COPPER, IODINE, IRON, MAGNESIUM, MANGANESE, PHOSPHORUS, POTASSIUM, SELENIUM, ZINC; FIBRE; PROTEIN; OMEGA-6 AND -9 ESSENTIAL FATTY ACIDS

These tiny seeds can add both taste and essential nutrients to a variety of sweet and savoury dishes. A fantastic source of calcium, sesame seeds are brilliant non-dairy bone-builders.

Sesame seeds have a nutty flavour and are slightly crunchy in texture to eat. Valuable health-boosters, they are made into a number of products, such as sesame oil, which is highly resistant to rancidity, and tahini, a sesame-seed paste, or simply scattered over stir-fries, salads and pasta.

Rich in zinc and antioxidant vitamin E, sesame seeds are powerful immunity boosters. They also contain a host of B-vitamins to support the nervous system and to help the body to cope with stress, as well as selenium to stave off wrinkles and keep the skin looking youthful. The seeds and oil are rich in calcium and magnesium – two important minerals, which are necessary for bone and heart health.

A good source of vegetarian protein, sesame seeds are packed with omega-6 fatty acids for healthy skin and hair, while sesame oil contains omega-9 fatty acids, which offer great benefits to the heart by reducing the risk of atherosclerosis and lowering cholesterol levels. Omega-9s also help to balance blood-sugar levels and enhance immunity.

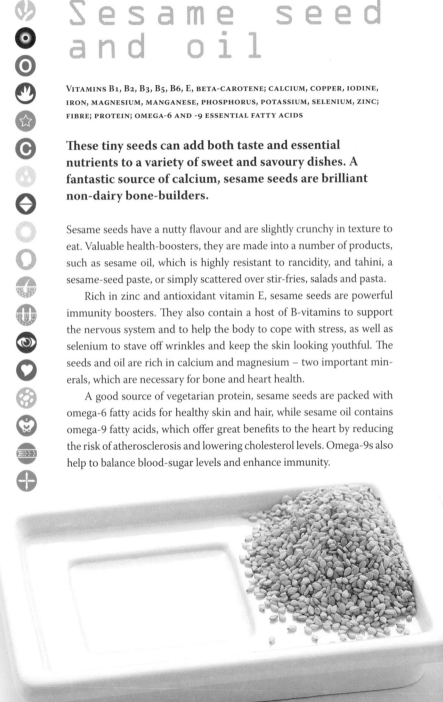

CRUNCHY SESAME STIR-FRY

3 tbsp olive oil

25g/1oz sesame seeds

2.5cm/1in root ginger, peeled and grated

2 garlic cloves, crushed

½ broccoli head, broken into small florets

3 carrots, peeled and cut into long thin slices

½ cabbage, cored and shredded

In a wok, heat the oil and sesame seeds until the seeds start to toast. Then add the ginger and garlic, followed by the other ingredients. Combine well. Turn the heat down to low, fry for a further 5–10 minutes and serve.

SESAME TAHINI DIP

350g/12oz/1¼ cups sesame seeds

4 tbsp groundnut oil

roasted vegetable pieces, to serve

Preheat the oven to 180°C/350°F/gas mark 4. Sprinkle the sesame seeds on to a baking sheet and toast in the oven for 20 minutes. Whizz the seeds in a blender for about 3 minutes, then add 1 tablespoonful of the oil and whizz for 30 seconds before adding the remaining oil. Whizz again until a smooth paste is formed. Serve with roasted vegetable pieces.

SESAME CHEWS

175g/6oz/1 cup dried dates

55g/2oz/½ cup chopped pecan nuts

2 tbsp tahini

2 tbsp peanut butter

4 tbsp sesame seeds

Put 250ml/9fl oz/1 cup water and the dates in a pan and simmer, covered, for 10 minutes until soft and the liquid is absorbed. Mash the dates and mix together with the pecan nuts, tahini and peanut butter. Allow to stand for about 30 minutes so that the mixture firms up, then form into small balls and coat with the sesame seeds.

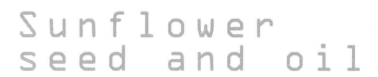

Sunflower seed and oil

VITAMINS B1, B2, B3, B5, E, FOLIC ACID; CALCIUM, COPPER, IRON, MAGNESIUM, MANGANESE, PHOSPHORUS, SELENIUM, ZINC; OMEGA-6 ESSENTIAL FATTY ACIDS; PROTEIN

Power-packed with a whole host of nutrients, sunflower seeds are one of the finest energy "pick-me-ups" that nature provides. Although small, they are loaded with life-enhancing antioxidants.

Sunflower seeds are a valuable source of B-vitamins, which means they are nourishing to the adrenal glands and thus may help to combat energy slumps and many symptoms associated with stress.

Sunflower seeds are a diuretic and expectorant, and have been used in the treatment of bronchial, throat and lung infections. The seeds and oil are full of vitamin E, omega-6 essential fatty acids and monounsaturated fats, which help to keep the skin elastic and minimize heart disease. Omega-6s also help to fight inflammation, so relieving arthritis. The essential fatty acid content may be beneficial in treating eczema.

The seeds and oil are rich in the minerals calcium and magnesium, needed for the contraction of muscles as well as a healthy bone structure. Magnesium is used in producing energy and calming allergic reactions. Sunflower seeds and oil also contain immunity-boosting zinc, a powerful antiviral, and selenium, which has potent antioxidant properties to fight the free radicals that harm the body's cells.

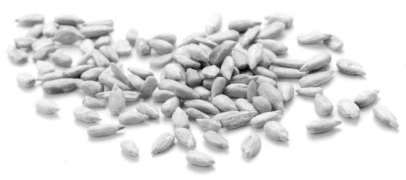

SUNFLOWER SEED OAT BREAD
makes 2 small loaves

500g/1lb 2oz/5 cups oat flour
6g/¼oz instant dried yeast
2 tbsp sunflower seeds
1 tsp salt
2 tbsp malt extract
400ml/14fl oz/scant 1⅔cups warm water
1 tbsp sunflower oil

Preheat the oven to 180˚C/350˚F/gas mark 4. Put the flour, yeast, seeds, salt and malt extract in a bowl and mix well. Add the water and oil. Form a dough. Knead for 10 minutes; divide into 2 and place in loaf tins. Cover and leave for 30 minutes. Bake for 50–60 minutes until browned.

SUNFLOWER SEED TOPPING

1 tbsp groundnut oil
4 tbsp sunflower seeds
1 tbsp sesame seeds
2 tbsp walnut halves
1 tbsp soy sauce
2.5cm/1in piece root ginger, peeled

Heat the oil in a wok until very hot. Add the seeds and walnuts, and fry for 30 seconds, stirring constantly. Add the soy sauce, then transfer to a bowl. Chop and add the ginger. Serve sprinkled on rice or stir-fries.

MUESLI

125g/4½oz/1¼ cups rolled oats
2 tbsp dried dates, chopped
2 tbsp dried apricots, chopped
1 tbsp pecan nuts, chopped
1 tbsp flaked almonds,
1 tbsp sunflower seeds
1 tbsp flaxseeds
1 tbsp wheatgerm
1 tbsp wheat bran
2 apples, peeled, cored
   and chopped
unsweetened soya milk,
   to serve

Combine all the dry ingredients in a bowl and top with the apple. Serve with the soya milk.

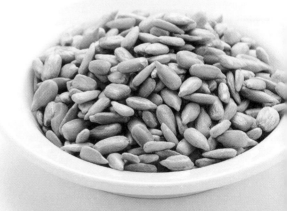

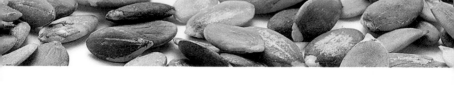

Pumpkin seed

VITAMINS B2, B3, B5, E, K, BETA-CAROTENE; CALCIUM, COPPER, IRON, MAGNESIUM, MANGANESE, PHOSPHORUS, POTASSIUM, SELENIUM, ZINC; OMEGA-3 AND -6 ESSENTIAL FATTY ACIDS

Tasty pumpkin seeds are full of essential fatty acids and many health-enhancing micronutrients. Boasting the highest iron content in the seed world, they make a very nutritious nibble.

Packed with nutrients, pumpkin seeds are full of omega-3 fatty acids, which are anti-inflammatory and so protect joints from damage and also promote the healing of sports-related injuries. Along with omega-6 fatty acids in the seeds, they are crucial for good immune function, as well as for healthy skin, blood clotting, digestion and nerve function. The essential fatty acids (EFAs) are also vital for youthful skin and glossy hair.

The EFAs in pumpkin seeds boost memory and are central to a healthy brain. Studies show that they can boost children's brainpower and are important for babies in the womb to avoid the risk of developing eye and nerve problems.

Pumpkin seeds may help to fight cardiovascular and immuno-deficiency disorders. The seeds are one of the richest natural sources of phytosterols, plant compounds that reduce the risk of arteries becoming narrowed by cholesterol. Phytosterols are also thought to boost immunity and have anti-carcinogenic properties.

The seeds are also rich in B-vitamins, which are vital for moderating stress and its damaging effects on the immune system. These vitamins play an important role in converting carbohydrates into energy as well as being essential for cell reproduction, which makes them beneficial for the tissues that grow and renew themselves, such as the hair and nails.

Pumpkin seeds contain many health-giving minerals including the antioxidants selenium and zinc, which support the immune system, helping to fight off diseases and infections. Selenium helps to neutralize the damaging effects of harmful free radicals and is thought to have anti-cancer activity. Owing to their high zinc content, pumpkin seeds have a reputation as a male sexual tonic and studies have shown that they can also help to reduce an enlarged prostate gland. A combination of zinc and essential fatty acids has been found to be particularly effective in combating prostate problems.

Pumpkin seeds are a good source of calcium and magnesium, which are needed for healthy bones, nerves and muscles. The magnesium ensures that the calcium is properly absorbed in the body. They also provide a valuable source of energy through the presence of digestible iron, which encourages the formation of red blood cells and helps to ensure that oxygen is pumped around the body efficiently, making fatigue and low energy levels during exercise less likely. Exercise requires good circulation, and pumpkin seeds are rich in a compound that could help. Pumping oxygenated blood rapidly around the body puts pressure on the arteries, which need to remain flexible and clear.

The seeds also make an effective dewormer and have been used to help to treat roundworm, tapeworm and other intestinal parasites.

PUMPKIN FRITTERS *serves 2*

1 small pumpkin, peeled and sliced

175g/6oz/scant 1 cup plain wholemeal flour

½ tsp salt

½ tsp baking powder

2 tsp ground cumin

1 egg, separated

185ml/6fl oz/¾ cup water

1 onion, chopped

2 garlic cloves, crushed

2 tbsp olive oil

2 tbsp hulled pumpkin seeds

Steam the pumpkin for 10 minutes, then leave to cool. In a bowl, combine the flour, salt, baking powder and cumin, then add the egg yolk and the water, a little at a time, stirring to form a smooth paste. Add the onion and garlic, then whisk the egg white and fold it in. Heat the oil in a frying pan, then dip the pumpkin slices in the mixture and fry a few at a time, turning until crisp and brown. Sprinkle with the seeds and serve.

PUMPKIN, PARSNIP AND CARROT SOUP

250g/8oz pumpkin, peeled and deseeded
250g/8oz parsnips, peeled
250g/8oz carrots, peeled
1 tbsp olive oil
15g/½oz butter
1 onion, chopped
900ml/34fl oz/3½ cups chicken or
  vegetable stock
1–2 tbsp lemon juice
2 tbsp hulled pumpkin seeds

Chop the vegetables. Heat the oil and butter in a pan and fry the onion until soft. Add the pumpkin, parsnips and carrots, and stir well. Cover, and cook for 5 minutes. Add the stock. Bring to the boil, cover and simmer for 30 minutes. Leave to cool, then blend until smooth. Reheat in the pan, add lemon juice to taste, then sprinkle with the pumpkin seeds and serve.

SEEDED MUFFIN CRUNCH

400g/14oz/3¼ cups plain flour
2 tsp baking powder
200g/7oz/1⅔ cups raisins
100g/3½oz/½ cup pumpkin seeds
2 carrots, peeled and grated
4 free-range eggs, beaten
200ml/7fl oz/¾ cup maple syrup
200ml/7fl oz/¾ cup milk
200ml/7fl oz/¾ cup sunflower oil

Preheat the oven to 180°C/350°F/gas mark 4. Combine the flour, baking powder, raisins and seeds in a bowl. Then, add the remaining ingredients and mix well to form a batter. Spoon the mixture into an oiled muffin tray and bake for 20 minutes or until the muffins are a light golden colour. Turn out on to a wire rack to cool.

PUMPKIN SEED PORRIDGE

300g/10½ oz/1½ cups pumpkin seeds
500–750ml/16–24fl oz/2–3 cups milk
clear honey, to taste

Grind the pumpkin seeds in a food processor or mill. Add 2 cups of milk and blend to form a porridge consistency. Add additional milk, as desired. Transfer to a pan and bring to the boil. Add honey to taste, and serve.

GREEK PEAR DESSERT *serves 2*

2 pears, chopped
200gl/7oz/heaped ¾ cup Greek yogurt
3 tbsp pumpkin seeds
1 tbsp sunflower seeds
1 tbsp manuka honey

Divide the chopped pears between two bowls and top with the yogurt. Sprinkle the seeds in a layer over the yogurt, then drizzle over the honey and serve.

PUMPKIN SEED BRITTLE

60g/2¼oz/⅓ cup sugar
60ml/2fl oz/⅔ cup water
100g/3½ oz/½ cup pumpkin seeds, toasted
1 tsp olive oil
a pinch of salt

Preheat the oven to 130°C/250°F/gas mark 1. Toss the pumpkin seeds in a bowl with the oil and a pinch of salt. Then, spread them evenly on a baking sheet in the middle of the oven for 1 hour, stirring occasionally. In a frying pan, combine the sugar and water, stirring continuously over a low heat, until the mixture is a deep caramel colour. Add the seeds, and stir until well coated. Turn out on to a greased sheet of foil. Leave to cool completely and break into pieces.

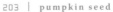

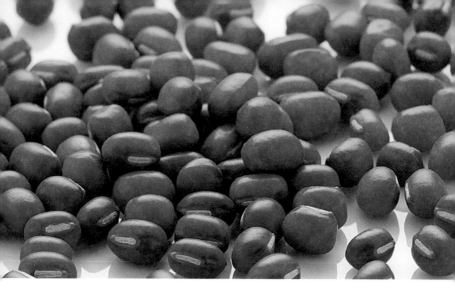

TASTY, VERSATILE AND
NUTRIENT DENSE, GRAINS,
PULSES AND BEANS FORM
THE CORNERSTONE OF
A HEALTHY DIET THE
WORLD OVER

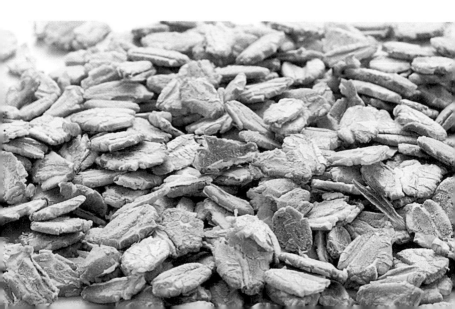

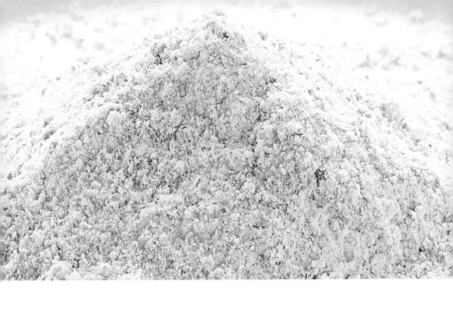

06 | **wonder**
GRAINS,
PULSES'
& BEANS

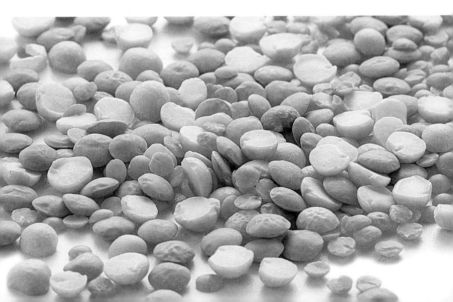

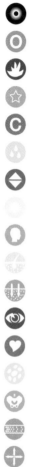

Wheat and wheatgerm

VITAMINS B1, B2, B3, B5, B6, E, FOLIC ACID; IRON, MAGNESIUM, MANGANESE, SELENIUM, ZINC, OMEGA-6 FATTY ACIDS, CHOLINE; PYRODOXINE; PROTEIN, FIBRE

A staple food in the Western diet, wheat is protein-rich, providing B-vitamins and minerals. The sprouting part of wheat grain, wheatgerm, is a super source of free-radical-fighting vitamin E.

Whole wheat is a nutritious and healthy cereal grain. A valuable source of protein, it provides important constituents for youthful skin, hair and nails. It also provides a valuable source of energy, thus combating fatigue. Whole wheat is rich in B-vitamins, including B6, which maintains the nerves, prevents adult-onset diabetes and also enhances the ability to register, retain and retrieve information. The grain is a good source of zinc, which boosts immunity and aids eye health.

Found inside the wheat grain, wheatgerm is the heart of the cereal, containing many of its most valuable nutrients. It is rich in the antioxidant vitamin E, which helps to detoxify the body by neutralizing harmful free radicals and has been shown to help to prevent heart disease. The high vitamin E content is especially good for keeping hair glossy and skin glowing. Wheatgerm is a very high-fibre food, and so helps to ensure an efficient digestive system, as well as to reduce cholesterol levels.

Used topically, wheatgerm's slightly granular texture gently exfoliates sensitive or dry skin.

Wholemeal bread and flour contain wheat germ. But it is missing from white bread and standard baking products, which is why these provide a quick energy rush that is followed by a slump.

HONEY WHEATGERM SMOOTHIE *serves 1*

200ml/7fl oz/scant 1 cup soya milk
55g/2oz/¼ cup plain bio-yogurt
125g/4½oz/scant 1 cup strawberries,
  hulled
1 large banana
2 tsp wheatgerm
2 tsp manuka honey

Whizz all the ingredients together in a blender and serve immediately.

SIMPLE WHOLEMEAL PIZZA CRUST

540g/1lb 3oz/4 cups wholemeal flour
2 tbsp dried yeast
1½ tsp salt
500ml /17 fl oz/2 cups warm water
2 tbsp extra virgin olive oil
2 tsp clear honey
topping of choice

Preheat the oven to 400°F/200°C/gas mark 6. Combine the flour, yeast and salt in a bowl. Add the water, oil and honey, and mix well. Cover with a moist cloth and leave to rise in a warm place for 10 minutes. Knead and press into a greased large pizza pan. Add the topping. Then, bake for 15–20 minutes.

*WHEATGERM LOTION *for exfoliating the skin*

250ml/9fl oz/1 cup milk
85g/3oz/1 cup dried chamomile
4 tbsp clear honey
2½ tbsp wheatgerm

Pour the milk into a cup and add the chamomile. Leave to infuse for a few hours. Strain the liquid and discard the chamomile. Add the honey and wheatgerm, and mix well. Pour the lotion into a bottle and store in the fridge for up to a week. Apply to the face and neck, then rinse off with warm water. Use as needed.

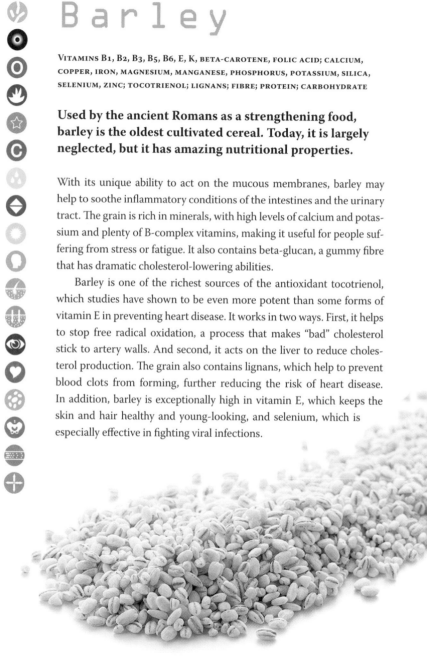

Barley

VITAMINS B1, B2, B3, B5, B6, E, K, BETA-CAROTENE, FOLIC ACID; CALCIUM,
COPPER, IRON, MAGNESIUM, MANGANESE, PHOSPHORUS, POTASSIUM, SILICA,
SELENIUM, ZINC; TOCOTRIENOL; LIGNANS; FIBRE; PROTEIN; CARBOHYDRATE

Used by the ancient Romans as a strengthening food, barley is the oldest cultivated cereal. Today, it is largely neglected, but it has amazing nutritional properties.

With its unique ability to act on the mucous membranes, barley may help to soothe inflammatory conditions of the intestines and the urinary tract. The grain is rich in minerals, with high levels of calcium and potassium and plenty of B-complex vitamins, making it useful for people suffering from stress or fatigue. It also contains beta-glucan, a gummy fibre that has dramatic cholesterol-lowering abilities.

Barley is one of the richest sources of the antioxidant tocotrienol, which studies have shown to be even more potent than some forms of vitamin E in preventing heart disease. It works in two ways. First, it helps to stop free radical oxidation, a process that makes "bad" cholesterol stick to artery walls. And second, it acts on the liver to reduce cholesterol production. The grain also contains lignans, which help to prevent blood clots from forming, further reducing the risk of heart disease. In addition, barley is exceptionally high in vitamin E, which keeps the skin and hair healthy and young-looking, and selenium, which is especially effective in fighting viral infections.

✦LEMON BARLEY WATER
for cystitis, constipation & diarrhoea

125g/4oz/⅔ cup pearl barley
1l/35fl oz/4 cups water
grated zest of 1 lemon
clear honey, to taste

Bring the pearl barley to the boil in a pan with 240ml/9fl oz/1 cup of the water. Strain, then add the remaining water and the lemon zest. Simmer until the barley is soft, adding water as required. Strain the liquid, sweeten with honey and leave to cool. Drink or keep in the fridge for up to 4 days.

✦BARLEY LOTION *to improve blood circulation*

100g/3½oz/½ cup pearl barley,
  soaked for 24 hours in cold water
1l/35fl oz/4 cups water
1 generous handful fresh rosemary or
  3 tbsp dried rosemary

Put the barley in a pan with the fresh water. Bring to the boil, cover and simmer for 30 minutes. Strain and discard the barley. Add the rosemary, cover and leave to infuse until cool. Strain into a glass bottle. Using cotton wool, apply twice daily. Store in the fridge for up to 4 days.

BARLEY AND VEGETABLE SOUP

55g/2oz/¼ cup pot barley, soaked
  overnight in cold water
2 tbsp olive oil
1 onion, chopped
1 garlic clove, crushed
2 celery sticks, trimmed and chopped
1 tomato, chopped
1 tbsp paprika
55g/2oz green beans, chopped
1.5l/52fl oz/6 cups vegetable stock
1 tsp dried mixed herbs

Drain the barley and put it in a large pan. Add all the other ingredients, then bring to the boil and simmer, covered, for about 1 hour.

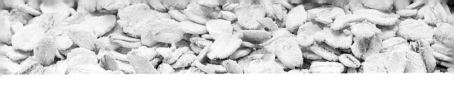

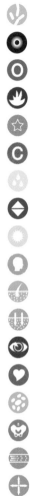

Oats

Vitamins B1, B2, B3, B5, B6, E, K, biotin, folic acid; calcium,
copper, iron, magnesium, manganese, phosphorus, potassium,
selenium, silica, zinc; saponins; tocotrienol, ferulic acid, caffeic
acid; flavonoids; fibre; protein; complex carbohydrate

Comforting and sustaining, oats bring a host of health benefits. For blood sugar maintenance, sustained energy and staving off hunger, there's no better breakfast than a steaming bowl of delicious porridge oats.

Although wild oats are thought to have originated in the Near East, domsticated oats first appeared in Europe in the Bronze Age. Today the grain is particularly suited to the cool wet summers of north-west Europe, where it is particularly popular.

Oats can be used in several ways, including being "rolled" to make a commercial foodstuff or kiln dried, stripped of their husks and delicate outer skins and then coarsely ground to make oatmeal or finely ground to constitute oat flour.

A cornucopia of nourishment, oats are a good source of protein, and are incredibly high in calcium, potassium and magnesium, which, like the B-vitamins, act as a nerve tonic, as well as promoting strong bones and teeth, and can aid weight loss because they release energy slowly, staving off hunger pangs. Oats have plenty of silica, which is anti-inflammatory and helps to maintain healthy arterial walls, as well as to keep nails strong and hair glossy. Their selenium and zinc increase the body's immune system and the ability to fight off infectious diseases.

These remarkable grains are also rich in fibre and singularly digest-ible, as well as having a demulcent quality that protects the duodenal surfaces, stomach and intestines. Oats are especially good for irritable bowel syndrome as they are anti-spasmodic.

High in immunity-boosting vitamin E, oats contain flavonoids called avenanthramides – potent antioxidants that help to break down choles-terol build-up and are thought to help prevent cancer, especially colon cancer. Other powerful, youth-promoting antioxidants found in oats include tocotrienol, ferulic acid and caffeic acid to fight against free radicals and protect against everything from heart disease to obesity and eye disease. Oats also have a mild tranquillizing effect, and boost mood, making them the perfect comfort food.

Research shows that oats can be helpful in staving off heart disease, diabetes and strokes. Eaten regularly, all kinds of whole grains are associated with good health in older people, but oats have special qualities. They contain a form of fibre called beta-glucan, which has an exceptional ability to reduce cholesterol – cutting the risk of strokes and heart disease from blocked arteries – and to stabilize blood sugar. Oats are a complex carbohydrate with a very low glycaemic index (GI). They therefore provide sustainable energy, alleviating insomnia and improving insulin sensitivity in people with diabetes.

As well as being the prime ingredient in porridge, oats are a mainstay of other breakfast cereals, such as muesli and granola. They are also used in a variety of baked goods, such as oat bread, oat cakes, flapjacks and oatmeal biscuits. Oat milk is now widely available as a drink and makes a useful alternative to cow's milk for people who are lactose-intolerant.

Used topically, oats have an emollient and anti-inflammatory effect on the skin, which makes them a common ingredient in beauty preparations. They can be used as a skin cleanser and exfolliant to remove the surface layer of dead skin cells. Oats are also found in bars of soap and when combined with water in the bath, they can help to alleviate and soothe skin irritations.

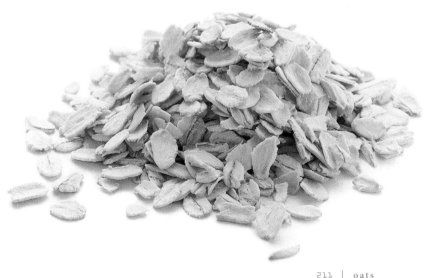

*OATMEAL HERBAL SCRUB *to cleanse the skin*

160ml/5¼fl oz/⅔ cup boiling water

3 tbsp dried parsley, lemon balm or
  fennel seeds

1 tbsp ground oatmeal

2 drops almond oil

Make a herbal infusion by pouring the water over the herbs and covering for 15 minutes. Strain and discard the herbs. Allow the infusion to cool, then add enough to the oatmeal to form a paste-like consistency. Add the almond oil. Smooth the scrub on the face and neck and leave for 20 minutes. Then, rinse off with tepid water and pat dry.

OAT CAKES

100g/3½oz/¾ cup fine oatmeal

a pinch of bicarbonate of soda

a pinch of salt

1 tbsp olive oil

Preheat the oven to 180°C/350°F/ gas mark 4. Mix together the oatmeal, bicarbonate of soda and salt. Add the oil and 2 tablespoons hot water and mix well to form a firm dough. Roll out on a floured surface. Cut into 8 rounds and place on a greased baking tray. Bake for 8–10 minutes until browned. Serve.

RAISIN FLAPJACKS

300g/10½oz/3 cups porridge oats

100g/3½oz/¾ cup raisins

150g/5½oz margarine

8 tbsp/½ cup clear honey

6 tbsp fruit sugar

1 tbsp natural vanilla extract

Preheat the oven to 190°C/375°F/ gas mark 5. Put the oats and raisins in a mixing bowl and set aside. Melt the margarine in a pan, add the remaining ingredients and stir. Pour onto the oats and mix well. Press into a non-stick baking tray, and cook for 15–18 minutes.

✦ OATEN JELLY *for gastric problems*

65g/2½oz/½ cup oat flour
450ml/16fl oz/2 cups water
15g/½oz butter
sugar or honey, to taste

Blend the oat flour with a little water. Boil the rest of the water in a pan and slowly pour onto the flour, stirring until thick. Return the mixture to the pan and add the butter. Bring to the boil and simmer for 7 minutes, stirring continuously, until thick. Add sugar or honey.

FRUITY PORRIDGE *serves 2*

850ml/29fl oz/3¼ cups unsweetened
* soya milk*
150g /5½oz/1½ cups porridge oats
1 tsp ground cinnamon
1 small banana, chopped
200g/7oz/1⅓ cups blueberries
2 tbsp flaked almonds

Put the soya milk and oats in a pan and cook over a low heat, stirring regularly, for 5 minutes. Add the cinnamon and banana, stir, and cook for 2 minutes. Divide the mixture into two bowls. Serve topped with the blueberries and flaked almonds.

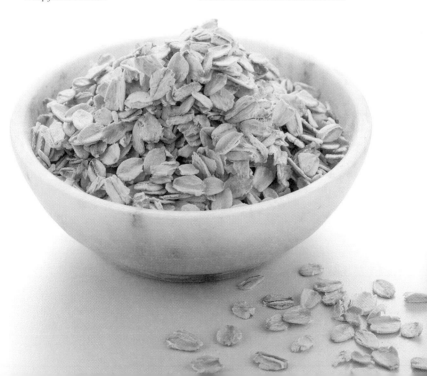

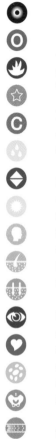

Quinoa

VITAMINS B1, B2, B3, B5, B6, E, FOLIC ACID; CALCIUM, COPPER, IRON, MAGNESIUM, MANGANESE, PHOSPHORUS, POTASSIUM, ZINC; FIBRE; PROTEIN; SAPONINS; CARBOHYDRATE

Pronounced "keenwa", and introduced from the South American Andes, quinoa is rich in unique health-sustaining properties, packed with goodness.

Known as the "mother grain" by the Incas, these bead-shaped grains are often called the "perfect food". This is because quinoa is a complete protein, containing all eight essential amino acids – an extremely rare quality in the plant world. Quinoa contains significantly more protein than other grains, making it especially useful for children and anyone suffering from anaemia or muscular degeneration. It is also particularly rich in the amino acid lysine, which the body needs to grow and repair tissue.

Quinoa contains a good range of B-vitamins, including B1, which is essential for the efficient functioning of the nervous, cardiovascular and muscular systems, and vitamin B2, which controls the build-up of cholesterol in the body by destroying harmful free radicals. Among the other B-vitamins found in quinoa are B5, which is essential for a healthy response to stress, and folic acid, which aids the reproductive organs and is crucial for the healthy production of red blood cells.

The grain is a useful source of antioxidant vitamin E, needed for the body's healing processes and to keep the skin youthful, as well as a number of health-enhancing minerals, including calcium, iron, manganese, magnesium and zinc. Calcium, magnesium and manganese are all vital for strong bones and for staving off osteoporosis, while iron helps to prevent fatigue, as well as hair loss and anaemia. Magnesium is also thought to play a role in averting migraines and headaches, and in lowering blood pressure. Zinc is a powerful antioxidant mineral that fights infections and is also necessary for the health of the thymus gland – the regulator of immune cell production.

In Eastern medicine, quinoa is used to strengthen the kidneys and revitalize the liver, as well as for everything from reproductive health and urinary problems to detoxification and skin disorders.

QUINOA PILAFF

850ml /29fl oz/3¼ cups water
350g /12oz/1¾ cups quinoa
150ml/5fl oz/scant ⅔ cup olive oil
450g/1lb okra, thinly sliced
3 tbsp tomato purée
1 onion, chopped
2 garlic cloves, crushed
2 tsp cumin seeds
1 tsp black pepper
55g/2oz coriander, chopped

Boil the water in a saucepan. Add the quinoa, bring to the boil again and simmer for 15 minutes. Drain. Heat the oil in a wok, add the okra and stir-fry for 3 minutes. Add the remaining ingredients apart from the coriander, and stir-fry for 5 minutes. Lower the heat and cook for a further 10 minutes. Mix in the quinoa and coriander. Serve.

SOUTH-WESTERN QUINOA AND CHICKPEA SALAD

90g/3¼oz/½ cup quinoa
500ml/17fl oz/2 cups water
4 tsp olive oil
225g/8oz/1 cup canned chickpeas, drained
1 tomato, deseeded and chopped
3 tbsp lime juice
2 tbsp chopped coriander
½ tsp ground cumin
1 garlic clove, finely chopped
a pinch of salt

Bring the quinoa and water to the boil in a pan, reduce the heat, cover and simmer for 15 minutes. Drain and transfer the quinoa to a bowl. Drizzle with the oil and toss. Add the remaining ingredients and mix well.

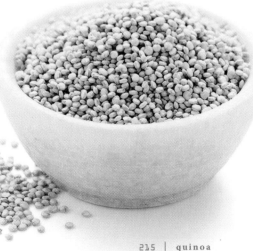

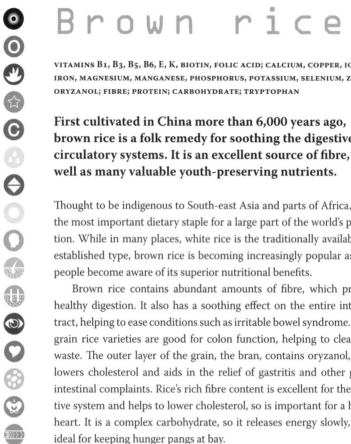

Brown rice

VITAMINS B1, B3, B5, B6, E, K, BIOTIN, FOLIC ACID; CALCIUM, COPPER, IODINE,
IRON, MAGNESIUM, MANGANESE, PHOSPHORUS, POTASSIUM, SELENIUM, ZINC;
ORYZANOL; FIBRE; PROTEIN; CARBOHYDRATE; TRYPTOPHAN

First cultivated in China more than 6,000 years ago, brown rice is a folk remedy for soothing the digestive and circulatory systems. It is an excellent source of fibre, as well as many valuable youth-preserving nutrients.

Thought to be indigenous to South-east Asia and parts of Africa, rice is the most important dietary staple for a large part of the world's population. While in many places, white rice is the traditionally available and established type, brown rice is becoming increasingly popular as more people become aware of its superior nutritional benefits.

Brown rice contains abundant amounts of fibre, which promote healthy digestion. It also has a soothing effect on the entire intestinal tract, helping to ease conditions such as irritable bowel syndrome. Short-grain rice varieties are good for colon function, helping to clear toxic waste. The outer layer of the grain, the bran, contains oryzanol, which lowers cholesterol and aids in the relief of gastritis and other gastro-intestinal complaints. Rice's rich fibre content is excellent for the digestive system and helps to lower cholesterol, so is important for a healthy heart. It is a complex carbohydrate, so it releases energy slowly, and is ideal for keeping hunger pangs at bay.

Dense in B-vitamins, brown rice is good for keeping the brain and nervous system healthy, and helps to relieve anxiety, fatigue and depression. Its protein is a building block for the bones and muscles, as well as soft tissues such as the skin and the hair. Brown rice is also a good source of trace minerals, such as phosphorus and copper, which build resistance to infections. Brown rice is also rich in magnesium, which plays a major role in bone health as well as reducing mood swings and easing stress, lowering high blood pressure, preventing muscle cramps and helping the body to turn food into energy. Containing iron to combat anaemia and hair loss, brown rice is also high in zinc, which is antiviral and excellent for warding off colds.

Many of the nutrients that could improve mood more effectively are lost when rice is processed to become white. Brown rice still contains all its nutrients and provides selenium, which counters depression but is lacking in most people's diets. Brown rice takes longer than white varieties to digest, preventing a sudden rise and fall in blood-sugar levels and making you feel comfortably full. It also makes a wonderful convalescing food as it is gentle on the stomach. Packed with phytonutrients, it is particularly useful in countering mood swings and other symptoms associated with the perimenopause.

According to the macrobiotic philosophy, brown rice is considered to be the most balanced of all foods and people who follow this dietary regime often eat it on a daily basis.

The processing of wholegrain rice into white rice removes many of its key nutrients and all of its fibre. So although brown rice takes longer to cook than white rice – about 45 minutes as opposed to 15 minutes – it's well worth the extra time. Brown basmati rice is not rapidly absorbed into the body, providing a steady stream of energy for exercisers, rather than a spike followed by a slump.

BROWN RICE SALAD *serves 1–2*

55g/2oz/¼ cup brown rice, cooked
  and cooled
2 spring onions, trimmed and sliced
4 tomatoes, cut into segments
100g/3½oz/½ cup black olives, pitted
  and halved
2 garlic cloves, crushed
3 tbsp basil, roughly chopped
3 tbsp olive oil

Combine all the ingredients together in a large salad bowl. Leave at room temperature for 1 hour to allow the flavours to mingle, then serve.

PILAU RICE

1 onion, finely chopped
1 tbsp olive oil
2 cardamom pods
5 cloves
½ cinnamon stick
a pinch of saffron threads
200g/7oz/1 cup brown basmati rice
800ml/28fl oz/3¼ cups vegetable stock
2 bay leaves

Sauté the onion in the oil until soft. Add the spices and cook for a further 2 minutes. Then add the rice and stir until the grains are coated in the oil before adding the stock and bay leaves. Bring to the boil, then simmer, covered, for about 50 minutes or until the rice is soft and all the liquid has been absorbed.

✦ GROUND RICE POULTICE
for skin inflammation

40g/1½oz/¼ cup ground brown rice
60ml/2fl oz/¼ cup milk
gauze or cotton strip

In a bowl, mix the rice and milk to make a paste. Apply to the affected area. Bandage securely in place, using the gauze or cotton strip. Leave on for up to 3 hours, as required.

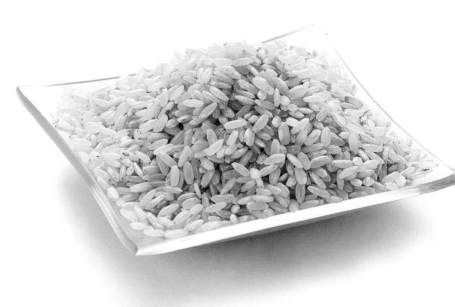

SPICED BROWN RICE

1l/35fl oz/4 cups water

300g/10½oz/1½ cups short-grain
   brown rice

600ml/21fl oz/2½ cups soya milk

4 tbsp rice syrup or date syrup

1 tsp ground cinnamon

¼ nutmeg, grated

4 cloves

2 small handfuls raisins

4 shavings orange zest

Preheat the oven to 180°C/350°F/gas mark 4. Put the water in a pan and bring to the boil. Add the rice and simmer for 15 minutes. Strain and return the rice to the pan. Add the remaining ingredients and simmer for 20 minutes. Turn into a lightly greased dish. Bake for 40 minutes.

RAISIN RICE PUDDING

300g/10½oz/1½ cups brown rice

4 tbsp raisins

250ml/9fl oz/1 cup milk

2 tbsp clear honey

2 tsp cinnamon

Boil the rice for 15 minutes, until tender. Preheat the oven to 160°C/ 325°F/gas mark 3. Mix the rice and raisins in a baking dish. In a pan, gently heat the milk and honey. Pour over the rice and sprinkle with cinnamon. Bake for 30 minutes and serve.

COCONUT MILK RICE PUDDING

200g/7oz/1 cup short-grain brown rice

3 tbsp raisins

2 tbsp agave syrup

1 cinnamon stick

10 cardamom pods

400ml/14fl oz/1⅔ cups coconut milk

½ tsp natural vanilla extract

ground cinnamon, to serve

Put the rice, raisins, agave syrup, cinnamon stick and cardamom in a pan with 1l/35fl oz/4 cups water and bring to the boil. Simmer, covered, for 90 minutes until the water is absorbed. Add the coconut milk and vanilla extract. Cook for 5 minutes. Sprinkle with the ground cinnamon and serve.

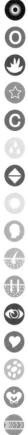

Buckwheat

Vitamins B1, B2, B3, B5, B6, E, K, folic acid; calcium, copper, iron, magnesium, manganese, phosphorus, potassium, selenium, zinc; rutin; chiro-inositol; fibre; protein; carbohydrate

This unique-tasting grain blends well when mixed with other grains and is marvellous for strengthening blood vessels and improving a sluggish circulation.

Thought to have originated in China, buckwheat spread to northern Europe and Russia in the fourteenth century. In spite of its name, buckwheat is not related to wheat and is suitable for those on a wheat- or gluten-free diet.

Buckwheat's main asset is its rutin, a bioflavonoid compound that helps to strengthen weakened blood capillaries, thus preventing the formation of thread veins. In turn, the strenthening of capillaries may improve circulatory problems such as chilblains and high blood pressure. Buckwheat also appears to aid the management of diabetes and glucose intolerance by controlling blood-sugar balance through the action of a substance called D-chiro-inositol.

Buckwheat contains fibre and all eight essential amino acids, and is a good source of protein for the brain. Rich in magnesium, which is vital for bone health, the grain also contains several B-vitamins, which help to maintain the nervous system. It also lowers blood cholesterol levels.

Buckwheat is today widely consumed in Eastern Europe, especially in Poland and Russia, where it features in many traditional dishes.

BUCKWHEAT MUESLI

200g/7oz/2½ cups buckwheat flakes
100g/3½oz/⅓ cup oats
50g/1¾oz/½ cup sunflower seeds
50g/1¾oz/1 cup dried apricots
50g/1¾oz/⅓ cup raisins
milk or soya milk, to serve

Chop the apricots into bite-sized pieces. In a large mixing bowl, combine the ingredients thoroughly. The muesli keeps well in a sealed plastic container. Serve with milk or soya milk.

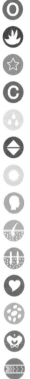

Millet

MAGNESIUM, POTASSIUM, SILICA; PROTEIN

Millet is a highly nutritious grain that supplies fantastic support to the digestive system, especially the stomach, spleen and pancreas.

Grown in Asia and Africa for thousands of years, millet was one of the first cereals to be cultivated by mankind. It is even mentioned in the Bible. Today, millet is gaining in popularity in the West.

High in protein, low in starch and containing all eight essential amino acids, millet is one of only a few alkaline-forming grains, so helping to counteract over-acidity in the stomach and joints. It has anti-fungal and anti-mucus properties, which help to prevent ailments such as candida and premenstrual discomfort.

Millet is rich in silica, the great cleansing, mending and eliminating mineral that is essential for hair, skin, teeth, eye and nail health, as well as the growth and maintenance of tendons and bones. Silica also supports arterial health, prevents cardiovascular disease and plays an important role in memory function. The grain has high levels of potassium and magnesium, useful for treating arthritis and osteoporosis.

MILLET PILAFF

1 large onion, finely chopped
4 tsp olive oil
2 tbsp ground coriander
2 garlic cloves, crushed
250g/9oz/2 cups millet
600g/1lb 5oz tomatoes, chopped
600ml/21fl oz/2½ cups vegetable stock
250ml/9fl oz/1 cup white wine
2 tsp flaked almonds
4–5 dashes of soy sauce

Preheat the oven to 180°C/350°F/gas mark 4. Gently fry the onion in oil for 4–5 minutes. Add the coriander and garlic, and fry for 5 minutes. Add the millet and cook for 2 minutes. Add the tomatoes, stock and wine. Bring to the boil, then simmer, uncovered, for 20 minutes until tender. Add the flaked almonds and soy sauce. Serve.

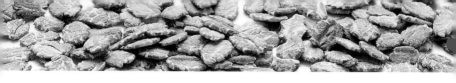

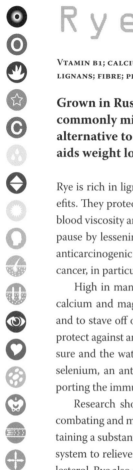

Rye

Vitamin B1; CALCIUM, IRON, MAGNESIUM, PHOSPHORUS, POTASSIUM, SELENIUM; LIGNANS; FIBRE; PROTEIN

Grown in Russia for more than 2,000 years, rye is commonly milled into flour and is used as a nutritious alternative to wheat. This high-fibre, low-GI cereal star aids weight loss and combats fluid retention.

Rye is rich in lignans, plant phytonutrients that have many health benefits. They protect against heart disease and stroke by helping to reduce blood viscosity and help women approaching or experiencing the menopause by lessening hot flushes and other symptoms. Lignans also have anticarcinogenic properties and are thought to prevent breast and colon cancer, in particular.

High in many health-enhancing minerals, rye is a useful source of calcium and magnesium, both of which are needed for healthy bones and to stave off osteoporosis. Its iron content helps to fight fatigue and protect against anaemia, while its potassium helps to control blood pressure and the water balance in the body's cells. Rye is also packed with selenium, an antioxidant mineral that plays an important role in supporting the immune system.

Research shows that rye is useful for balancing blood sugar and combating and managing diabetes, as it improves insulin response. Containing a substantial amount of dietary fibre, rye stimulates the digestive system to relieve constipation and is also thought to help to lower cholesterol. Rye also contains sucrose and fructooligosaccharide, which have prebiotic properties that are useful to digestive health.

Wholegrain cereals play an important role in weight loss. Full of insoluble fibre, they score low on the glycaemic index (GI), meaning they release sugar into the blood slowly, whereas refined versions have little nutritional value and cause a sudden spike in energy, then a slump. Low-GI foods have long been known to benefit health, but they are now thought to aid fat loss, too, even when you eat the same number of calories as on a higher-GI diet. Rye is one of the lowest GI cereals. It's also rich in compounds that bind food to water, which prevents bloating.

COTTAGE CHEESE ON RYE

8 slices of rye bread
8 tbsp/½ cup cottage cheese
1 tsp finely sliced lemongrass
4 tomatoes, roughly chopped
4 gherkins, sliced

Toast the bread. Mix together the cottage cheese and lemongrass. Pile onto the toast and top with the tomatoes and gherkins. Serve immediately.

RYE PANCAKES

100g/3½oz/½ cup rye flour
1 large egg
100ml /3½fl oz/½ cup water
150ml/5fl oz/scant ⅔ cup milk
1 tbsp olive oil

Whizz the rye flour, egg, water and milk in a food processor. Leave to stand for 10–15 minutes. Drizzle some oil into a heavy frying pan and heat. Carefully ladle in the batter, allowing 2–3 tablespoons per pancake. As the mixture for each pancake begins to bubble on the surface, flip it over and leave for 4–5 minutes or until cooked through.

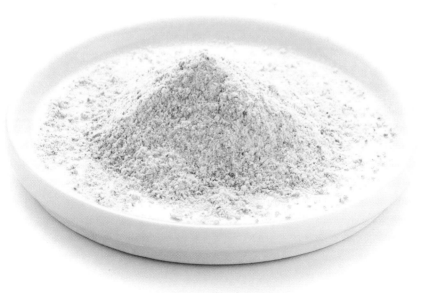

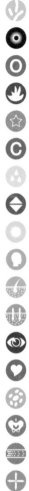

Soya bean

VITAMINS B1, B2, B3, B5, B6, E, K, BETA-CAROTENE, BIOTIN, FOLIC ACID;
CALCIUM, COPPER, IODINE, IRON, MAGNESIUM, MANGANESE, PHOSPHORUS,
POTASSIUM, SELENIUM, ZINC; FIBRE; PROTEIN; COMPLEX CARBOHYDRATE;
OMEGA-3 AND OMEGA-6 ESSENTIAL FATTY ACIDS; LECITHIN; ISOFLAVONES;
PHYTIC ACID, SAPONINS, PROTEASE INHIBITORS

Originating in Japan, soya beans are made into a number of food products with a wealth of ancient medicinal properties. Eating a diet rich in soya beans is believed to help to prevent heart disease, as well as to promote youthfulness and longevity.

Soya beans are the most widely grown beans in the world. They are available in many forms, including dried, tinned, fresh and frozen. Until recently they have perhaps been best known in Western countries in derivative products, such as soya milk, soy sauce and textured vegetable protein (TVP). However, the fresh beans are becoming increasingly popular, especially the young beans in their pods, known as edamame.

Unlike other legumes, soya is a source of complete protein, rivalling meat, fish and eggs, making it an ideal alternative for vegetarians, vegans and those who simply wish to reduce their consumption of meat. This versatile legume is central to the diet of the Japanese, who have the longest life spans in the world. Plant-derived protein is also said to help guard against gallstones.They are excellent in promoting healthy colon and bowel function, and are protective against constipation, diverticular disease and haemorrhoids.

Soya beans are an excellent source of dietary fibre and complex carbohydrates. They are known to have a cholesterol-lowering effect and to prevent high triglyceride levels, which can cause heart disease. In addition, soya beans contain youth-preserving antioxidants, such as phytic acid, which can help to prevent the clogging of the arteries that can lead to a stroke or a heart attack.

However, perhaps the most useful attribute of soya beans is that they are extremely rich in micronutrients, such as saponins and isoflavones. A type of flavonoid, isoflavones are converted by the body into phytoestrogens and have anti-carcinogenic properties as well as the ability to reduce the risk of cardiovascular disease and to promote bone health. The isoflavone genistein is thought to stop the breakdown of bone and to help to increase bone mass, offering protection against osteoporosis and it may also increase the flexibility of blood vessels. Phytoestrogens can also mimic the effects of the hormone oestrogen in the body. This makes them useful for helping to control menopausal symptoms, such as hot flushes. Studies have shown that isoflavones can help to prevent the hormone-linked diseases of breast and prostate cancer.

The beans contain vitamin E, which is vital for preserving youthful skin and hair, and B-vitamins, which maintain the nervous system and keep stress from causing premature aging.

Having an extremely low glycaemic index (GI) score, soya beans are great blood sugar and insulin regulators, which makes them useful for helping to prevent diabetes as well as for maintaining energy levels in people who already have the disease.

Soya beans are rich in lecithin, a natural emulsifier of fats, which helps them to assist in lowering cholesterol levels. Their omega-3 essential fatty acids stimulate blood circulation, reduce blood pressure and lower the risks of heart disease. Omega-3s also boost brain power, improve the quality of the skin and protect against cancer.

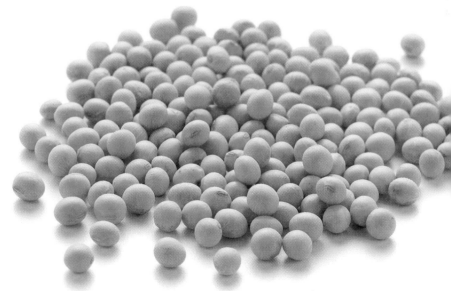

SOYA PANCAKES

125g/4½oz/1 cup soya flour
345g/12oz/2¾ cups plain flour
3 tbsp baking powder
3 tbsp sugar
½ tsp salt
3 eggs
750ml/24fl oz/3 cups soya milk
6 tbsp soya oil
a knob of butter

Combine all the ingredients, except the butter, in a bowl and beat to form a batter. Melt a little of the butter in a frying pan and add ½ cup of the batter. Cook on both sides until golden brown. Remove from the pan and keep warm while you cook the reamaining batter. Fold and serve.

BANANA, AVOCADO AND SOYA SMOOTHIE *serves 2*

1 banana, peeled
1 avocado, pitted and peeled
100g/3½oz silken tofu
400ml/14fl oz/1½ cups soya milk
a generous sprinkling of flaked almonds

Whizz together the banana, avocado, tofu and soya milk in a blender until smooth. Sprinkle over the flaked almonds and serve immediately.

SOYA BEAN PÂTÉ

200g/7oz/1 cup soya beans, cooked
1 tbsp olive oil
1 medium onion, finely chopped
2 tbsp tomato purée
10 black olives, pitted and chopped
2 tbsp chopped parsley
1 tbsp sesame seeds, lightly toasted
a pinch of salt

Put the soya beans in a bowl and mash them with a fork. Heat the olive oil in a frying pan and sauté the onion until it is clear and soft. Add to the beans. Stir in the tomato purée, olives, parsley, sesame seeds and salt. Chill for at least 30 minutes before serving.

SCRAMBLED TOFU

2 garlic cloves, crushed

½ large red pepper, deseeded and diced

2 tbsp olive oil

300g/10½oz firm tofu

½ tsp ground turmeric

½ tsp salt

pinch of ground black pepper

1 onion, chopped

1½ tsp soy sauce

salsa and corn tortillas, to serve

In a frying pan, sauté the garlic and red pepper in the olive oil for 2 minutes. Crumble the tofu and add to the pan, then add the turmeric, salt, black pepper, onion and soy sauce. Cook for 3 minutes, stirring occasionally. Remove from the heat. Serve with salsa and corn tortillas.

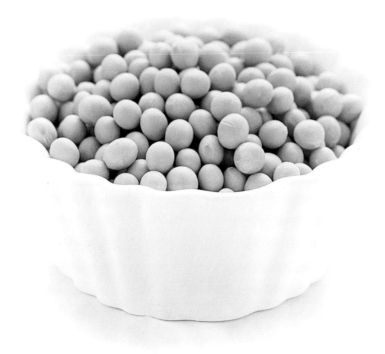

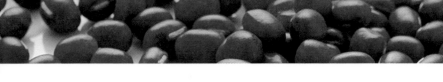

A d u k i   b e a n

Vitamins B1, B2, B3, B5, B6, E, beta-carotene, biotin, folic acid; calcium, copper, iodine, iron, magnesium, manganese, phosphorus, potassium, selenium, zinc; fibre; protein; carbohydrate

These nutty beans, known as the "king of beans" in Japan – where they have been used for their healing properties for more than 1,000 years – are packed with energizing nutrients.

According to Oriental medicine, aduki beans help to disperse stagnant blood, which can be the cause of many diseases. They have a tonifying effect on the kidney-adrenal function and therefore help to regulate the stress response. Aduki beans are drying in nature, and are useful in the treatment of diarrhoea, oedema and boils. They are also good for the urinary tract and a drink made from the water in which aduki beans have been boiled is a traditional remedy for kidney and bladder complaints.

Aduki beans are high in fibre, making them useful for speeding up the elimination of waste and helping to detoxify the body. They contain good levels of B-vitamins, which are needed for steady energy production and to repair body tissues. Aduki beans are also a useful source of protein, which helps to build muscle and maintain healthy skin, and are rich in immunity-boosting minerals including antiviral zinc, calcium and magnesium.

They contain more fibre and protein and less fat than most other beans, making them useful for anyone trying to lose weight. They are diuretic and their high potassium content helps to control water balance by heping to rid the body of excess fluid.

ADUKI BEAN SOUP

200g/7oz/1 cup dried aduki beans
600ml/21fl oz/scant 2½ cups
   vegetable stock
1 onion, sliced
1 carrot, diced
1 celery stick, diced
soy sauce, to taste

Put all the ingredients, except the soy sauce, in a pan. Bring to the boil, then simmer for 1 hour, or until the vegetables are tender. Add the soy sauce to taste. Blend in a food processor if desired.

ADUKI BEAN CHILLI

100g/3½oz/½ cup dried aduki beans
1 onion, chopped
1 clove garlic, crushed
2 tbsp olive oil
400g/14oz tin chopped tomatoes
½ green chilli, deseeded and finely chopped
½ tsp chilli powder
1 tbsp tamari

Soak the beans overnight in cold water. Next day, drain, put in a pan with water and bring to the boil. Simmer, covered, for about 1 hour until soft. Drain and set aside. In another pan, gently fry the onion and garlic in the oil, add the remaining ingredients and the beans, and simmer, covered, for 25 minutes.

ADUKI BEAN HOTPOT

100g/3½oz/½ cup dried aduki beans
1 large onion, chopped
3 carrots, peeled and diced
2 parsnips, peeled and diced
2 sweet potatoes, peeled and diced
2 bay leaves
1 tbsp tomato purée

Soak the beans overnight in cold water. Drain, put in a pan and cover with water. Bring to the boil, reduce the heat and simmer for 45 minutes. Drain. Put all the ingredients into a large casserole dish with water to cover. Bake in a pre-heated oven at 190°C/375°F/gas mark 5 for 1½ hours.

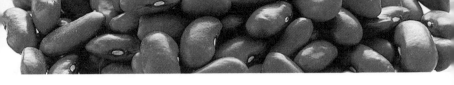

Kidney bean

VITAMINS B1, B6, K, FOLIC ACID; COPPER, IRON, MAGNESIUM, MANGANESE, MOLYBDENUM, PHOSPHORUS, POTASSIUM, ZINC; FIBRE, PROTEIN

Thought to originate from Peru, these soft beans are high in protein, vitamins and minerals. This small but powerful food provides an armoury of nutrients to keep mind and body on top form.

Popular in Central and South America, kidney beans are an excellent source of protein, which helps to keep energy levels steady as well as maintaining and repairing cells. One average serving of kidney beans provides lots of protein and one third of the recommended daily intake of fibre. This is beneficial for regular exercisers who want to lose weight, because fibre curbs hunger for longer, while the protein gives energy. The soluble fibre keeps blood-sugar levels steady, giving you plenty of vitality while preventing energy spikes and slumps. This means that these beans are especially useful for people with diabetes or hypoglycaemia, too. Fibre also protects the heart and cardiovascular system by lowering blood cholesterol, and it encourages good digestion and the efficient elimination of toxins and waste matter.

The humble kidney bean provides an impressive array of nutrients for combating low moods and strengthening brain function. Rich in vitamin B1, it keeps the memory sharp and its rich magnesium content promotes physical and mental relaxation. Kidney beans contain iron – crucial for the production of the immune system's antibodies and white blood cells. They also provide an iron top-up for the many women whose periods leave them short of this essential mineral.

Kidney beans are also rich in folic acid, a B-vitamin that is important for good reproductive health, especially in early pregnancy for protecting the developing foetus from spina bifida. Folic acid also combats heart disease and helps to speed up wound healing.

QUICK KIDNEY BEAN CASSEROLE *serves 2*

2 tbsp olive oil

1 onion, chopped

1 red pepper, deseeded and chopped

1 courgette, sliced

4 Portabello mushrooms, sliced

270g/9½ oz/1½ cups tinned kidney beans

3 large tomatoes, chopped

2 garlic cloves, crushed

2 tsp chopped basil

1 tsp salt

Heat the olive oil in a large saucepan, then add the onion and stir-fry until golden. Add the pepper, courgette, mushrooms, tomatoes and garlic, stir for 5 minutes, then add the kidney beans, and enough water to cover. Add the basil and salt, then cover and simmer until the vegetables are soft.

KIDNEY BEAN GUMBO

1 red onion, chopped

1 red pepper, deseeded and diced

1 celery stalk, trimmed and chopped

2 garlic cloves, crushed

1 tbsp olive oil

1.5l/52fl oz/6 cups vegetable stock

425g/15oz/1½ cups chopped tomatoes

1 tsp dried thyme

a pinch of cayenne pepper

270g/9½ oz/1½ cups tinned kidney beans

In a saucepan, fry the onion, red pepper, celery and garlic in the oil for 5 minutes. Add the stock, tomatoes, thyme and cayenne pepper, cover and simmer until soft. Add the kidney beans and simmer for 10 minutes. Serve.

CHILLI BEANS

1 tbsp groundnut oil

2 onions, chopped

1 tsp chilli powder or 1 fresh chilli, deseeded and chopped

225g/8oz lean minced beef (optional)

270g/9½ oz/1½ cups tinned kidney beans

400g/14oz/1⅔ cups tinned tomatoes

Heat the oil in a pan and fry the onions for 2–3 minutes. Add the chilli powder and fry for 1 minute. Stir in the beef, if using, and cook until browned. Add the beans and tomatoes and bring to the boil. Reduce the heat and simmer for 10 minutes. Serve with brown rice.

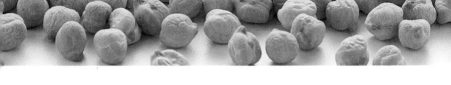

Chickpea

VITAMINS B1, B2, B3, B5, B6, E, K, BETA-CAROTENE, BIOTIN, FOLIC ACID; CALCIUM, COPPER, IODINE, IRON, MAGNESIUM, MANGANESE, MOLYBDENUM, PHOSPHORUS, POTASSIUM, SELENIUM, ZINC; FIBRE, PROTEIN, CARBOHYDRATE

Grown from the equatorial tropics to the temperate northern latitudes of Russia, chickpeas are a popular staple that rates among the most nutritious of pulses.

Packed with health-enhancing nutrients, chickpeas are a good source of isoflavones – plant chemicals that are converted in the gut into a substance that mimics the hormone oestrogen. They can therefore help to prevent hormone-related conditions including PMS and breast cancer. Chickpeas have antiseptic properties and are a diuretic, making them useful to combat cystitis and oedema. They also aid the absorption of nutrients and are good for digestive health. In addition, chickpeas support the functions of nerves and muscles in the body as well as helping to stabilize blood sugar.

Chickpeas are loaded with protein, which is vital for the healthy repair of cells. They also contain protease inhibitors, which halt the DNA-destroying action of cancer cells. They are rich in antioxidant vitamin E, which promotes the ability of white blood cells to fight infection, protects the heart and promotes healthy skin and hair. They contain zinc, which enhances immunity and rejuvenates the thymus gland. Chickpeas

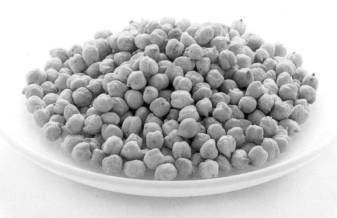

also provide plenty of iron, a mineral that women in particular, tend to be deficient in until after the menopause.

It is thought that chickpeas also help the body to deal with preservatives, found in some fast foods, that can cause headaches. Tinned chickpeas (without added sugar or salt) are just as nutritious as dried.

CHICKPEA SALAD

225g/8oz/1½ cups dried chickpeas
10 spring onions, trimmed and sliced
200g/7oz watercress
200g/7oz rocket leaves
1 handful chopped mint
3 tbsp olive oil
2 tbsp balsamic vinegar
115g/4oz/1 cup Parmesan shavings

Soak the chickpeas overnight. Drain, place in a pan and cover with water. Bring to the boil, reduce the heat and simmer for 2 hours until soft. Once cool, mix well with the onions, watercress, rocket, mint, oil and vinegar in a large bowl. Scatter over the cheese and serve.

HUMMUS

400g/14oz/2¼ cups tinned chickpeas
2 garlic cloves, crushed
3 tbsp lemon juice
2 tbsp tahini
2 tbsp olive oil

Drain the chickpeas and blend with the garlic and lemon juice, or mash them in a bowl. Stir in the tahini and oil, and add a little water for smoothness, if wished.

CHICKPEA CURRY

150g/5½oz/⅔ cup chickpeas, soaked in
    water overnight
1 onion, chopped
2 garlic cloves, crushed
2 tsp curry powder
2 tbsp olive oil
500ml/17fl oz/2 cups passata

Drain the chickpeas and put in a pan with water. Bring to the boil and simmer, covered, for 2 hours. Drain and set aside. Sauté the onion, garlic and curry powder in the oil. Add the passata and chickpeas, and simmer, covered, for 25 minutes. Serve.

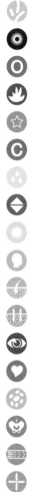

Lentil

VITAMINS B1, B2, B3, B5, B6, B9, B12, E, K, BETA-CAROTENE, BIOTIN, FOLIC ACID; CALCIUM, COPPER, IODINE, IRON, MAGNESIUM, MANGANESE, PHOSPHORUS, POTASSIUM, SELENIUM, ZINC; FIBRE; PROTEIN; CARBOHYDRATE

The humble lentil, one of our oldest foods and a staple in many countries, is antioxidant-rich and one of the single most nutritious and digestible foods of all.

Whether red, green or brown, lentils are a good source of protein, which we need to keep our skin, hair, teeth and nails strong and healthy. They contain high levels of B-vitamins, particularly B3, deficiency of which can lead to poor memory and irritability, and B12, which helps to prevent everything from arthritis to tinnitus. Along with the antioxidant selenium, the B-vitamins also help to boost the body's immune system, aiding the fighting of bacteria and other invaders. They are rich in iron and are recommended for pregnant and lactating women, as well as people suffering from anaemia. As with all other pulses, lentils contain anti-carcinogenic phytochemicals and are also a good source of plant oestrogens, which can help to reduce menopausal symptoms.

Lentils are loaded with fibre, which promotes a healthy digestive system and can help to regulate colon function as well as boosting heart-health and the circulatory system. They are great for stabilizing blood-sugar levels, making them a useful food for diabetics.

Providing the perfect combination of nutrients to allay hunger pangs and spark energy, lentils are an ideal snack to have before exercising or playing sports. A spoonful of dhal on bread, for example, is sustaining but not heavy, so it won't slow you down or cause indigestion. Lentils are rich in complex carbohydrates, which the body turns into glucose, providing a steady source of energy to maintain stamina. In fact, one study found that eating lentils three hours before exercise could help to increase endurance significantly more than other carbohydrates. They also contain very little fat.

Lentils are crammed full of folic acid, an energy-boosting vitamin that plays a key role in the production of serotonin, the neurotransmitter in the brain associated with feelings of happiness.

SPICY LENTIL BURGERS

1 onion, finely chopped
1 tbsp olive oil
1–2 tsp curry powder
175g/6oz/scant 1 cup red lentils
450ml/16fl oz/scant 2 cups vegetable stock
125g/4oz/1 cup wholemeal breadcrumbs

Fry the onion in the oil, then stir in the curry powder and cook for 2 minutes. Add the lentils and stock. Bring to the boil, then simmer for 20–25 minutes. Add the breadcrumbs and shape into four burgers. Grill on a lightly oiled baking tray until crisp and brown.

WARM LENTIL SALAD

300g/10½oz/heaped 1 cup red lentils
50ml/2fl oz olive oil
2 onions, chopped
1 garlic clove, crushed
1 red pepper, deseeded and finely chopped
1 courgette, finely chopped
1 carrot, peeled and finely sliced
1 celery stick, finely chopped
2 large ripe tomatoes, deseeded and
  chopped
2 tbsp balsamic vinegar
1 tbsp finely chopped mint

Cook the lentils in a pan in boiling water for 30 minutes or until tender, then drain. Heat the oil in a wok, add the vegetables and stir-fry until tender. Remove from the heat, add the lentils, vinegar and mint, combine thoroughly, and serve.

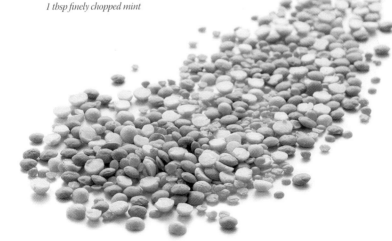

SWEET AND SOUR LENTILS

250g/9oz/1 cup red lentils
2 tbsp vegetable oil
2 dried red chillies, chopped
½ tsp mustard seeds
2 tbsp soy sauce
1 tbsp sugar
4 tbsp pineapple juice
1 tbsp white wine vinegar

Place the lentils in a pan, cover with water and bring to the boil. Cover the pan, reduce the heat and simmer for 40 minutes; drain. In another pan, heat the oil and spices for 3 minutes. Add the soy sauce, sugar, juice, vinegar and lentils. Stir in 125ml/ 4fl oz/½ cup water, simmer for 10 minutes, then serve.

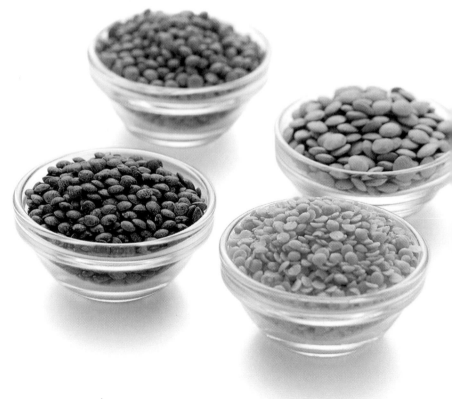

LENTIL AND CUMIN SOUP

2 onions, roughly chopped

4 garlic cloves, crushed

4 tsp cumin seeds

3 tbsp vegetable oil

1 bay leaf

½ tsp dried oregano

3l/104fl oz/12 cups chicken stock

600g/1lb 5oz/3 cups tinned green or
brown lentils

In a saucepan sauté the onion, garlic and cumin seeds in the oil. Add the bay leaf, oregano and stock. Bring to the boil, then reduce the heat and simmer for 10 minutes. Add the lentils and cook for a further 10 minutes. Remove the bay leaf and purée the soup in a food processor.

DHAL

1 tbsp groundnut oil

1 tsp mustard seeds

1 large onion, finely chopped

2 garlic cloves, crushed

1 tsp ground cumin

2.5cm/1in piece root ginger, peeled and
finely chopped

200g/7oz/¾ cup lentils

Heat the oil and fry the mustard seeds until they pop. Add the onion, garlic, cumin and ginger and stir-fry for 3–5 minutes until the onion is softened. Add the lentils and 750ml/26fl oz/3 cups water and bring to the boil. Simmer for 30–40 minutes. Serve with bread or rice, or refrigerate overnight.

RED LENTIL DHAL

2 tbsp olive oil

1 onion, chopped

2 garlic cloves, crushed

1 tsp ground mustard seeds

1 tsp ground cumin

½ tsp chilli powder

½ tsp turmeric

2 tomatoes, chopped

200g/7oz/¾ cup red lentils

Heat the oil in a pan and gently fry the onion until soft. Add the garlic, spices and tomatoes and simmer for a few minutes, stirring. Add the lentils and 500ml/17fl oz/2 cups water, and bring to the boil, then reduce the heat and simmer, covered, for 20 minutes.

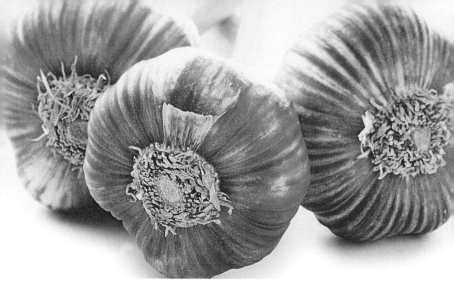

HERBS, SPICES AND
FOODS SUCH AS HONEY
AND CIDER VINEGAR
PUNCH WELL ABOVE
THEIR WEIGHT IN THE
NUTRITION STAKES

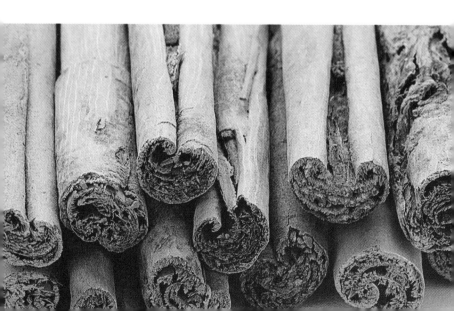

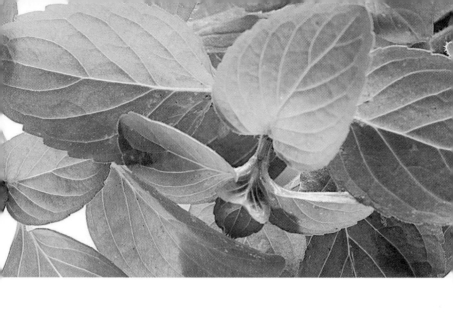

07 | wonder
HERBS,
SPICES
& OTHERS

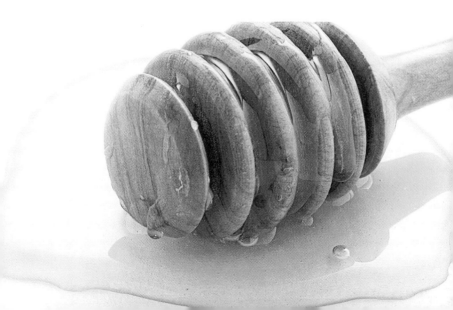

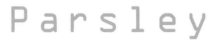

Parsley

VITAMINS A, B1, B3, B5, C, K, BETA-CAROTENE, BIOTIN, FOLIC ACID;
CALCIUM, COPPER, IODINE, IRON, MAGNESIUM, MANGANESE, PHOSPHORUS,
POTASSIUM, SELENIUM, ZINC; LIMONENE, MYRISTICIN; LUTEOLIN

One of the world's most popular culinary herbs, parsley has much more to it than its use as a garnish. Parsley is full of youth-enhancing nutrients and is a natural healer.

A great source of disease-fighting antioxidants, parsley is high in vitamin A and its precursor, beta-carotene, as well as vitamin C. Vitamin A is known for its ability to keep the arteries clear from the build up of plaque and for protecting against eye disease. It is a potent anti-inflammatory agent, which, along with vitamin C and the flavonoid luteolin, is thought to be useful in combating asthma and arthritis. Vitamin C fights the harmful free radicals that encourage the development of many diseases, such as cancer, diabetes and heart conditions. A powerful immunity-booster, vitamin C also staves off day-to-day illnesses, such as colds, flu and ear infections.

Parsley is the richest herbal source of the mineral potassium, which reduces high blood pressure – the number one cause of heart attacks. A natural diuretic, parsley encourages the excretion of sodium and water. Its potassium helps to balance fluid levels in the body, which can be disturbed by exercise, and also stimulates the kidneys to eliminate waste matter. Potassium is destroyed in cooking, so eat parsley raw to obtain maximum benefits.

The herb is also an excellent source of magnesium and calcium to protect the bones and the nervous system, as well as manganese, which boosts the memory, iron to prevent fatigue, and copper and zinc, which aid the healing of wounds.

Parsley contains several substances, including limonene, that exhibit anti-cancer properties, particularly against tumours. They also are believed to neutralize the carcinogens in cigarette smoke.

Chewing on a parsley sprig after a meal can help to freshen the breath. When applied topically to the skin, the herb is said to relieve irritation caused by insect bites.

PARSLEY SAUCE

25g/1oz butter
1 tbsp plain flour
400ml/14fl oz/1⅔ cups milk
2 tbsp double cream
juice and grated zest of ½ lemon
4 tbsp finely chopped parsley
ground black pepper

In a small pan, gently melt the butter, then stir in the flour to form a smooth paste. Gradually add the milk, bring the sauce to the boil, stirring all the time, then reduce the heat. Simmer for 3 minutes, whisking constantly. Add the cream, lemon juice and zest and parsley, and season with black pepper.

PARSLEY PASTA SAUCE

2 tbsp olive oil
½ onion, chopped
1 garlic clove, crushed
1 tsp paprika
400ml/14fl oz/1⅔ cups passata
3 tbsp chopped parsley
salt and ground black pepper

Heat the oil in a pan and gently fry the onion until soft. Add the garlic and paprika and continue to cook for 1 further minute, stirring. Add the passata and simmer, covered, for 20 minutes. Add the parsley and seasoning toward the end of cooking time. Serve over pasta.

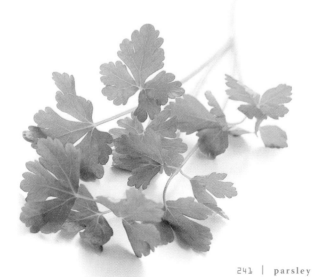

Sage

VITAMINS B3, B6, C, E, K, BETA-CAROTENE, BIOTIN, FOLIC ACID; CALCIUM, IRON, MAGNESIUM, MANGANESE, PHOSPHORUS, POTASSIUM, ZINC; FLAVONOIDS; TANNINS, SAPONINS, POLYPHENOLS; VOLATILE OILS

A native of the Mediterranean, this common garden herb is popular both used in cooking, and for its many curative properties.

With its rich array of nutrients, sage has antiseptic, anti-bacterial and anti-viral properties, and is a traditional ingredient of cough, cold and respiratory remedies. Sage is anti-mucosal, so it is useful for beating colds as it helps to clear catarrh as well as fight off germs, and it is particularly successful in the treatment of bronchitis. Its antiseptic properties make it excellent for healing gum problems and sore throats when drunk as a tea or used as a gargle, and its antioxidant and anti-inflammatory action can help to ease arthritis. It also clears sluggish skin and firms tissues.

Sage has several ways of improving mind and mood. Recent research has shown that the herb can increase brain power, particularly short-term memory – for example in word-recall tests. It contains compounds similar to those in drugs that are used to combat the formation of plaques in the brain, and research is now under way to find out if it can help to slow the progression of Alzheimer's disease. The herb is also thought to soothe emotional distress.

Thanks to its success in reducing perspiration, sage is now a popular remedy for hot flushes during the menopause. By preventing hot flushes and night sweats, it promotes healthy sleep patterns. Sage stimulates the intestines and is a digestive tonic. In Germany, it has been approved for the treatment of mild gastro-intestinal complaints. A sage infusion taken after eating can ease indigestion and bloating, as it is an anti-spasmodic herb.

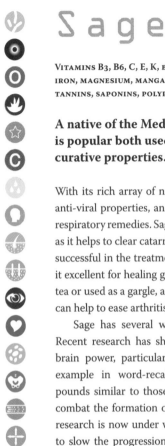

SIMPLE SAGE STUFFING

225g/8oz onions
115g/4oz/1½ cups fresh breadcrumbs
1 tsp dried sage
ground black pepper
25g/1oz butter, melted, plus extra for
  greasing

Preheat the oven to 200°C/400°F/gas mark 6. Quarter the onions and cook in boiling water until tender. Then drain and chop finely. Place in a bowl, mix in the breadcrumbs, sage and pepper, then add the melted butter to help the mixture stick together. Grease a baking tray and place scoops of mixture on it, then bake for 15 minutes. Suitable for serving with meat and vegetables.

✦ SAGE GARGLE *for respiratory ailments*

1 large handful sage leaves
1 small handful thyme leaves
450ml/16fl oz/scant 2 cups boiling water
2 tbsp cider vinegar
2 tsp clear honey
1 tsp cayenne pepper

Roughly chop the leaves and place in a jug. Add the boiling water, cover and leave for 30 minutes. Strain off the leaves and stir in the cider vinegar, honey and cayenne. Gargle with the mixture at the first sign of symptoms, or drink 2 teaspoons 2 or 3 times a day. Use within a week.

SQUASH SOUP WITH SAGE

450g/1lb deseeded and chopped squash
500ml/18fl oz/2 cups vegetable stock
1 tbsp olive oil
2 onions, chopped
4 tbsp chopped sage leaves
ground black pepper, to taste

Boil the squash for 10 minutes until tender. Place in a blender, add the stock and purée until smooth. Heat the oil in a pan. Sauté the onions for 3 minutes, adding half the sage for the last minute. Add the squash and bring to the boil. Reduce the heat and simmer for 10 minutes. Add the pepper and remaining sage. Serve.

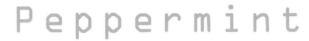

Peppermint

VITAMINS A, B2, B3, C, E, BETA-CAROTENE, FOLIC ACID; CALCIUM, COPPER, IRON, MAGNESIUM, MANGANESE, PHOSPHORUS, POTASSIUM; FIBRE; OMEGA-3 FATTY ACIDS; VOLATILE OILS

A well-known digestive aid, peppermint has many other benefits and is one of the most popular traditional remedies used today. This dark green, strongly flavoured variety of mint can help to beat colds and flu.

Native to Europe but now grown all over the world, peppermint is not a species in its own right but a hybrid of spearmint and watermint. Often known as the world's oldest medicine, peppermint may have been used as a remedy for more than ten thousand years.

Peppermint contains menthol, a substance useful for clearing congestion in the nose and chest from colds and infections. It is calming and anti-inflammatory, and also a good source of the minerals iron, needed for healthy blood, and calcium, necessary for strong bones and teeth.

This useful herb also improves the circulation, and can help to treat both chills and fevers. In addition it has analgesic properties, which are useful for headaches, inflamed joints, neuralgia and sciatica. The volatile oils are anti-bacterial, anti-parasitic, anti-fungal and anti-viral. They also have antiseptic qualities, which make it ideal for use in toothpastes and mouthwashes to protect teeth and gums, as well as to freshen the breath. Traditionally it has been used to treat toothache.

From a bunch of fresh leaves to a tube of sweets, any form of peppermint can relieve digestive upsets fast. It soothes the burning pain of indigestion, counteracts nausea, kills bacteria, relieves wind and regulates intestinal movement. Its ability to stop muscle spasm makes it a useful remedy for irritable bowel syndrome and for the abdominal cramps felt during painful periods. It has also been found to inhibit the growth of several types of bacteria, including *Helicobacter pylori*, which has been identified as being the main cause of stomach and duodenal ulcers. However, use it with caution if you suffer from heartburn (when stomach acids rise into the throat), as although peppermint helps many sufferers, others find that it makes their heartburn worse.

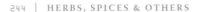

PIPERADE   *serves 1*

1 yellow pepper, deseeded and sliced

1 onion, sliced

3 tbsp olive oil

2 tomatoes, sliced

a pinch of cayenne pepper

1 tbsp finely chopped mint

1 egg

Fry the pepper and onion in the oil over a low heat until the onion is soft. Add the tomatoes, cayenne pepper and mint. Stir for 2 minutes, then break the egg over the vegetables and cook until the yolk is cooked as desired. Serve immediately.

✦PEPPERMINT FOOTBATH   *for tired feet*

50g/2oz peppermint leaves, roughly chopped

1 litre/35fl oz/4 cups boiling water

1.75l/44fl oz/7½ cups hot water

1 tsp borax

1 tbsp Epsom salts

Combine the herbs with the boiling water in a large bowl. Leave for 1 hour, then strain. Add to a bowl or footbath filled with the hot water. Stir in the borax and Epsom salts. Soak the feet for 15–20 minutes.

MINT TEA

4 tbsp finely chopped peppermint

2.5cm/1in piece root ginger, peeled and finely chopped

2 tsp clear honey

Boil 500ml/18fl oz/2 cups water and pour over the mint and ginger in a bowl. Leave to steep until cool enough to drink. Stir in the honey and drink when dissolved.

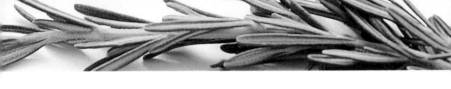

Rosemary

BETA-CAROTENE; CALCIUM, IRON, MAGNESIUM, MANGANESE; SAPONINS;
CAFFEIC ACID; FLAVONOIDS; VOLATILE OILS; FIBRE

This wonderfully fragrant and intensely flavoured herb has a range of health-enhancing properties. A potent, stimulating herb, rosemary is an old-fashioned remedy for everything from colds and colic, to nervousness, stress and eczema.

Rosemary has antiseptic, antioxidant, anti-spasmodic and astringent qualities, proving useful for circulatory conditions, stiff muscles, coughs and colds, mouth and gum infections, and irritable bowel syndrome. An invigorating herb, rosemary fights fatigue. It is also a nervine and is excellent for female complaints and headaches.

Rosemary has traditionally been prized for its ability to improve the memory, and it's not a myth: this herb can help to counteract a tendency to forgetfulness. A compound called rosmarinic acid improves blood circulation, increasing the flow of oxygen-rich blood to the brain. This improves all kinds of brain functions, aiding concentration and alertness. People perform better in memory tests, and have been found to be more alert, when they work in a room smelling of rosemary. And at the same time they also feel more relaxed and contented.

Recent studies on rosemary have shown that rosmarinic acid and another powerful antioxidant and anti-inflammatory agent known as caffeic acid may have the ability to help to prevent cancer. Current research shows that they may be particularly effective against breast cancer. The compounds also counter age-related skin damage such as wrinkles, as well as boost liver function and act as a mild diuretic. Together with vitamin E, they have significant abilities to fight the free radicals that cause premature aging and are thought to increase the risk of cancer.

Traditionally, rosemary essential oil has been used as an insect repellent. Applied topically, it helps to strengthen the blood capillaries and has a rejuvenating effect on skin and hair, making it a popular ingredient in many beauty products, including skin lotions, creams, toners, soaps and hair shampoos and conditioners.

✦TONIC WINE AND LINIMENT
for stiff muscles, headaches, etc.

1 handful rosemary leaves
2 small cinnamon sticks
5 cloves
1 tsp ground ginger
bottle of good-quality red wine

Lightly crush the rosemary, cinnamon and cloves in a tall jar, using a pestle. Add the ginger, then the wine, then seal the jar and leave in a cool place for 7–10 days. Strain and store in a sealed bottle. Drink a glass daily, or dip a cotton-wool pad in and apply to the affected area.

ROSEMARY POTATOES

450g/1lb potatoes, cut into wedges
2 tbsp groundnut oil
1 garlic clove, crushed (optional)
black pepper, to taste
1 tbsp chopped rosemary

Boil the potato wedges for 10 minutes until tender. Heat the oil and sauté the garlic and potatoes until the potatoes are browned and crunchy. Add the pepper and rosemary for the final minute of cooking time and serve immediately.

SOOTHING ROSEMARY TEA *makes 1 cup*

1 tsp dried rosemary
1 tsp dried marjoram
1 tsp dried feverfew
1 tsp dried peppermint

Mix the herbs well and place in a teapot. Add one cup of boiling water, and leave to infuse for 10 minutes, then strain and drink.

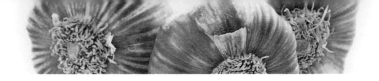

Garlic

VITAMINS B1, B3, B5, B6, C, BIOTIN, FOLIC ACID; CALCIUM, COPPER, GERMANIUM, IODINE, IRON, MAGNESIUM, MANGANESE, PHOSPHORUS, POTASSIUM, SELENIUM, SULPHUR, ZINC; AMINO ACIDS, S-ALLYLCYSTEINE, VOLATILE OILS; PROTEIN; FIBRE

An ingredient few cooks would be without, this pungent bulb has many therapeutic properties. Acclaimed as a superfood, garlic guarantees extra protection for over-worked joints and helps to keep the heart healthy, too.

Originally from Asia, garlic is part of the onion family. It was known in ancient Egypt and Greece, where it played a role in rituals as well as being an important medicinal food. Widely used today in cooking throughout the world, garlic is versatile and tasty, and can be added to virtually any savoury dish to boost its flavour – add one clove per person for its full health-boosting effects. It gives a kick to stir-fries, casseroles and sauces, and can be chopped and added raw to salads and dressings. For those who find the taste of garlic overpowering, it can also be taken in supplement form.

Known for its powerful smell and taste, garlic's protective powers are even stronger, ranging from fighting cancer to promoting weight loss. Its most potent properties stem from a rich supply of compounds containing sulphur, which is what creates that distinctive smell. The sulphur helps in the formation of new cells, keeping skin, nails and hair young-looking. It is also said to treat cellulite.

Garlic has been found to aid weight loss even if you make no other changes to your diet. It helps to make low-calorie meals more tasty, providing added flavour with virtually no calories. At the same time, it lowers blood levels of insulin, reducing the risk of weight-related problems such as metabolic syndrome and diabetes. Garlic doesn't just discourage your body from putting on weight from fats – even more importantly, it helps to prevent fatty deposits forming in your arteries, where they gradually harden and restrict

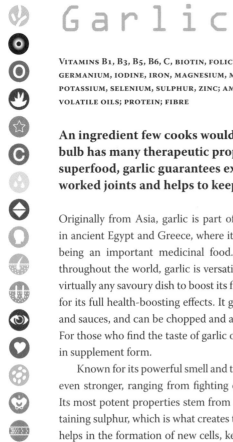

blood flow, and it lowers blood pressure. People who are trying to lose weight often eat high-protein diets and take extra exercise. These actions can result in an inflammatory response in the body, which can compromise immunity and reduce resistance to disease. In such cases, adding a clove of garlic a day to your diet has been proved to be very effective in counteracting inflammation.

Traditionally, garlic has been used to fight a range of diseases, from gastro-intestinal conditions to respiratory infections. A potent anti-microbial, garlic boosts the production of white blood cells and fights off bacteria, parasites, fungi and viruses. These properties make it a useful weapon against many conditions, from yeast infections to food poisoning and the common cold. It is also a powerful antioxidant, thanks to its amino acids, helping it to enhance overall immune function. This amazing food is useful for combating bladder and kidney problems, as well as ear infections. It also improves digestion and enhances the absorption of food.

Garlic contains a volatile oil called allicin, which is released when it is crushed, encouraging the elimination of cholesterol from the body, lowering triglyceride levels, detoxifying the liver and acting as a potent anti-inflammatory. It also inhibits blood-platelet stickiness, which is associated with the formation of blood clots, and heart attacks and strokes. In addition, garlic contains a compound called s-allylcysteine, which appears to have an anti-carcinogenic action. Ajoene, which is produced from allicin, may be useful in the treatment of skin cancer when applied topically. Other anti-cancer compounds in garlic include the powerful antioxidant minerals germanium and selenium.

✦ GARLIC SYRUP *for colds*

1 garlic bulb, cloves peeled and crushed
250ml/9fl oz/1 cup water
juice of ½ lemon
2 tbsp clear honey

Put the garlic and water in a pan, and bring to the boil. Reduce the heat and simmer for 10 minutes. Add the lemon juice and honey and simmer for a further 2–3 minutes. When cool, strain into a dark glass bottle. Take 2–3 tablespoons 3 times a day. Store in the fridge for 2–3 weeks.

GARLIC MUSHROOM SALAD

4 garlic cloves, crushed
12 large open mushrooms
3 tbsp olive oil
4 handfuls rocket leaves
115g/4oz feta cheese

In a pan, gently fry the garlic and mushrooms in the oil. Arrange the rocket leaves in 4 piles on four plates. Put three mushrooms on each pile, crumble over the feta cheese, and serve.

GARLIC-INFUSED OLIVE OIL

250ml/9fl oz/1 cup extra virgin olive oil
  (see method)
8 garlic cloves
1 tsp crushed dried chillies

Buy a 250ml/9fl oz bottle of extra virgin olive oil and add the whole garlic cloves and chillies. Some of the oil may have to be removed before infusing so that it doesn't spill over. Secure the lid and leave in a cool, dark cupboard for several days to allow the flavours to mingle. Use as required for cooking or as a salad dressing.

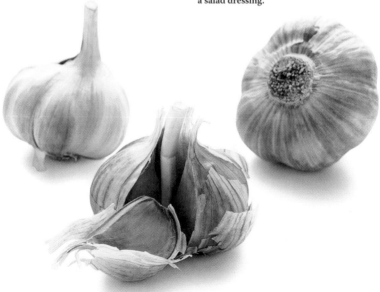

TOMATO, BASIL AND GARLIC SALAD

800g/1lb 12oz large tomatoes, sliced
4 tbsp roughly chopped basil
2 garlic cloves, finely chopped
6 tbsp olive oil
2 tbsp balsamic vinegar
salt and ground black pepper

Arrange the tomatoes flat on a large plate, and sprinkle over the remaining ingredients. Serve immediately.

GARLIC SOUP

2 tbsp olive oil
4 garlic cloves, crushed
200g/7oz/2 cups fresh breadcrumbs
1 litre/35fl oz/4 cups hot vegetable stock
4 eggs (optional)
crusty bread, to serve

Heat the oil in a pan over a low heat and sauté the garlic for about 30 seconds. Add the breadcrumbs and sauté for 1 minute. Stir in the stock, and bring to the boil, then simmer for 10 minutes. Break the eggs, if using, into the soup and poach for about 3 minutes. Serve with crusty bread.

REFRIED BEANS

250g/9oz/1¼ cups red kidney beans
3 tbsp olive oil
3 garlic cloves, crushed
1 tsp chilli powder
1 tsp ground cumin
1 tsp ground mustard seeds
1 tsp tamari

Soak the beans in cold water overnight. Drain, then put in a pan and cover with water. Bring to the boil, reduce heat and simmer, covered, for about 2 hours. Drain and set aside. Put the remaining ingredients with 100ml/3½fl oz/ ⅓ cup water in another pan and sauté for a few minutes. Add the beans and mix well. Mash until creamy.

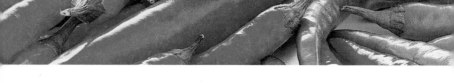

Chilli

VITAMIN C, BETA-CAROTENE; IRON, POTASSIUM, CAPSAICIN; FIBRE

According to traditional Oriental theory, "If you have a cold, you can build a fire in your stomach" with a spice such as chilli. These fiery hot peppers could also burn away some unwanted weight, as they boost metabolism and raise your temperature.

Even in small amounts, chillies are a helpful addition to the diet – one small red chilli contains high levels of the antiviral, anti-cancer and antioxidant carotenoid beta-carotene, some of which is converted into vitamin A in the body. Both these nutrients help to prevent the damage caused by toxins in the body, and can help to stave off cancer and premature aging. Chillies also contain capsaicin, a plant chemical that has natural analgesic properties, which can be used both internally and topically to ease headaches, arthritis and sinusitis.

According to Chinese medicine, chilli is a hot, pungent yang spice and a highly effective decongestant for colds as well as respiratory disorders. It flushes out the sinuses and clears the lungs, so treating various bronchial conditions. Chilli also acts on the circulatory and digestive systems, and is used to treat a wide range of complaints ranging from arthritis and chilblains to colic and diarrhoea.

Some experts say that chillies increase the body's fat-burning ability for about 20 minutes after a meal, so that you are literally burning up the food you've just eaten faster than normal. Others say that the fiery taste simply makes you eat more slowly, or that the tastiness makes food more satisfying. Whatever the reason, adding some of these hot peppers to your everyday diet does seem to aid weight control.

A recent Australian study seems to indicate that chillies could help diabetics, as they seem to significantly reduce the amount of insulin needed to lower blood-sugar levels after a meal. Chillies also alleviate chronic indigestion and kill the bacteria that cause stomach ulcers, though eating too many chillies is to be avoided, as research suggests it could increase the risk of stomach cancer.

ROAST CHILLI RELISH

200g/7oz chillies, deseeded
1 tbsp olive oil
4 garlic cloves, crushed
1 cucumber, finely chopped

Grill the chillies for 4–5 minutes until the skins blister. Put in a sealed plastic bag for 10 minutes. Rub the skins off and finely chop the chillies. Mix with the remaining ingredients. Keep in the fridge for up to 2 weeks. Use sparingly.

SPICY RICE *serves 2*

200g/7oz/1 cup long-grain rice
grated zest of 1 lime
1 garlic clove, peeled
1 red chilli, sliced
juice and grated zest of 2 lemons
1 tbsp wholegrain mustard
4 tbsp olive oil

Place the rice, lime zest and garlic in a pan, cover with water and bring to the boil, then simmer until the rice is tender. Drain and remove the lime zest and garlic. Combine the remaining ingredients in a bowl, then stir the mixture into the rice. Serve as a side dish.

✦ CHILLI PASTE *for colds & bronchial conditions*

3 small Thai dried chillies
2 garlic cloves, halved
1 small onion, chopped
30g/1oz sugar
3 tbsp lemon juice
3 tbsp water
½ tsp salt

Put the ingredients in a blender and whizz until finely chopped. Pour the mixture into a pan and cook gently, stirring occasionally, for 10 minutes. Makes 100ml/3½fl oz/ scant ½ cup of paste.

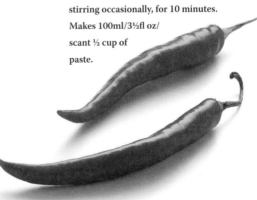

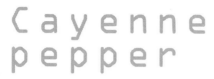

Cayenne pepper

VITAMINS A, B1, B3, B5, B6, C, CAROTENOIDS; CALCIUM, IRON, MANGANESE, POTASSIUM; CAPSAICIN; FLAVONOIDS, VOLATILE OILS, FIBRE

The name "cayenne" derives from the name of a town in French Guiana. A fiery spice, cayenne pepper is a variety of chilli, which was first introduced to the West in the sixteenth century.

A rich source of vitamins A and C, as well as many of the B-vitamins, cayenne pepper is useful for everything from eye health to immune function, and healthy skin to good memory. It is strongly anti-bacterial, can break down catarrh and has antioxidant properties that boost immunity and aid the body in fighting the damage caused by free radicals. Cayenne is also very high in calcium, which staves off osteoporosis, and potassium, which helps to regulate the body's fluid levels.

Its active constituent capsaicin is a warming stimulant and a powerful remedy for poor circulation, helping to dilate blood vessels and increase blood supply to all parts of the body. This makes it useful for people experiencing general debility and malaise, such as post-viral fatigue (ME) sufferers. Capsaicin, which also gives cayenne its antiinflammatory properties, has been widely studied for its pain-reducing effects and its ability to help to prevent stomach ulcers. .

Cayenne pepper also offers great cardiovascular benefits by helping to revitalize the veins and arteries so that they regain youthful elasticity. The pepper also strengthens the heart and regulates blood pressure, helping to prevent strokes and heart attacks.

Taken to relieve wind and colic and to stimulate secretion of the digestive juices, cayenne encourages the process of waste eliminination in the gut. It is also known to boost metabolism and to aid weight loss.

When applied topically to the skin, capsaicin desensitizes nerve endings and acts as a counter-irritant, helping local blood flow. It may help psoriasis, neuralgia, headaches and arthritis.

✳ CAYENNE-INFUSED OIL *for the skin*

100g /3½oz/scant 1 cup finely chopped
cayenne pepper
500ml/17fl oz/2¼ cup vegetable or
olive oil

Place the cayenne and oil in a heat-proof bowl. Bring a large pan of water to the boil, reduce the heat and simmer gently. Set the bowl over the pan and leave to simmer for 2–3 hours. Remove from the heat and allow to cool. Pour the infused oil, using a funnel, into a dark glass bottle. Apply to the skin as needed.

✦ WARMING CAYENNE WAX
to treat painful, inflamed joints

225g/8oz beeswax
2 cayenne peppers, or 1 dried cayenne
pepper
⅔ tsp St John's wort

In a pan, melt the beeswax and add the cayenne peppers. Simmer for 10 minutes, then remove the pepper. Stir in the St John's wort. Pour the warm mixture into empty ice cube trays and freeze. Melt 1 cube as needed. As it melts, lay out some paper tissue and, using a pastry brush, paint on the wax in a strip. Wrap the tissue strip around the painful area. To retain heat, cover the area in cling film. Leave on for 20 minutes. Repeat 3 times a week.

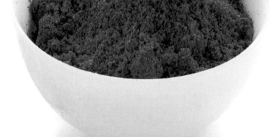

Turmeric

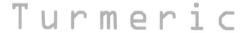

VITAMINS B3, B6, C, E, K, FOLIC ACID; CALCIUM, IRON, MAGNESIUM, MANGANESE, PHOSPHORUS, POTASSIUM, SELENIUM, ZINC; CURCUMIN

Grown for its root, which has a host of beneficial properties, turmeric is the most commonly used flavouring and colouring agent in Eastern cuisine.

Many spices would have stronger medicinal effects if they were not eaten in such small quantities. Turmeric, however, is such a potent anti-inflammatory that the small amount used in a curry is enough to reduce the risk of many illnesses and conditions.

Turmeric is used in traditional Chinese medicine to treat the liver and gallbladder. Elsewhere, it is a useful remedy that may help everything from gallstones and jaundice to premenstrual discomfort and skin conditions. It is also an anti-coagulant, and appears to prevent platelet stickiness, which helps to guard against heart disease and strokes.

The potent ingredient is curcumin, which gives turmeric its vivid golden colour. It has been shown to protect against inflammatory bowel disease and several forms of cancer , including prostate cancer and childhood leukemia. In addition, turmeric may counteract the carcinogenic effects of some additives that are found in processed food. Its anti-inflammatory properties are also very effective in relieving the pain and stiffness of arthritis and rheumatic problems.

Curcumin is a powerful antioxidant that is very effective at fighting free radicals and therefore protects the skin, eyes and hair, and keeps them youthful. It also has anti-bacterial and cholesterol-lowering properties. Research shows that curcumin may also protect against memory deterioration, and recent studies suggest that it may one day form the basis of a treatment for cystic fibrosis.

✦ TURMERIC POULTICE *for skin inflammation*

dried piece turmeric root

gauze bandage

Grind the turmeric in a blender to make a powder. Mix 1 teaspoon of the powder with a little water to make a paste. Wrap the paste in a gauze bandage and tie to the affected area. Leave for 20 minutes, then discard. Repeat 3 times a day.

SPICED CAULIFLOWER

1 large cauliflower, broken into florets

1 tbsp groundnut oil

1 tsp ground coriander

1 tsp ground black pepper

1 large onion, chopped

1 tsp salt

1 tbsp ground turmeric

Steam the cauliflower for 10 minutes. Meanwhile, heat the oil in a pan over a low heat and briefly fry the coriander and black pepper. Add the onion and stir-fry for 3–5 minutes until translucent. Add the salt and turmeric. Stir in the cauliflower until well coated and serve.

THAI CURRY SAUCE

400ml/14fl oz/1⅔ cups coconut milk

2 green chillies, deseeded and chopped

2 garlic cloves

2 tsp grated root ginger

1 tbsp olive oil

2 shallots, chopped

1 lemon grass stalk, peeled

1 tsp ground turmeric

2 tbsp chopped coriander

rice, to serve

Put the coconut milk, chillies, garlic and ginger in a blender and whizz. Heat the oil, add the shallots and fry gently until soft and golden. Add the coconut mixture and the remaining ingredients. Bring to the boil, reduce the heat and simmer for 5 minutes. Serve with rice.

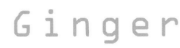

Ginger

Vitamins B3, B6, C, E, folic acid; calcium, copper, iron, magnesium, manganese, phosphorus, potassium, selenium, zinc; gingerol; phenols, volatile oil

Said to have derived from the Garden of Eden, ginger is a favourite spice and flavouring, and one of the world's greatest medicines. With its soothing, pain-relieving and anti-inflammatory properties, ginger is invaluable as a food remedy.

Used in India and China since 5000bc, ginger is grown throughout the tropics and used extensively as both a culinary and therapeutic spice. It contains an active constituent, gingerol, which has anti-cancer properties and is responsible for much of its hot, pungent taste and aroma, as well as its stimulating properties.

Ginger is useful for anyone feeling sluggish because it is stimulating and promotes detoxification by increasing perspiration and circulation. Recognized by scientists as a fast-acting cure for nausea of all kinds, it relieves complaints such as motion and morning sickness, reducing all associated symptoms, including dizziness and vomiting. Keeping ginger biscuits to hand during early pregnancy is a piece of advice that's been handed down for generations.

Ginger's volatile oil works on the digestive system by encouraging the secretion of digestive enzymes. Ginger is a wonderful remedy for indigestion, wind and colic. It protects the digestive system against premature aging, thus aiding the general absorption of nutrients. It also invigorates the stomach and intestines, easing constipation and removing the accumulation of toxins, including fungal infections, thus increasing vitality and well-being. The root helps to regulate blood sugar, both by stimulating pancreas cells and by lowering cholesterol levels.

Ginger is particularly rich in the mineral zinc – essential for a healthy immune system. The spice is warming and soothing, and is a favourite home remedy for colds and influenza. It promotes perspiration, reducing a fever and clearing congestion, and has a stimulating and expectorant action in the lungs, expelling phlegm and relieving coughs. It is a potent antiseptic. Ginger is also a useful remedy for pain and inflammation, helping cramps, peptic ulcers, allergies and asthma. Its gingerol, which suppress the substances that trigger joint pain and swelling, make it one of the most respected foods for the treatment of joint problems, such as osteoarthritis and rheumatoid arthritis.

Ginger has a stimulating effect on the circulation, lowering high blood pressure. Ginger supports heart health by preventing blood platelets from sticking together and lowering cholesterol levels, thereby offering protection against heart attacks and strokes.

To gain the strongest benefits, pour hot water on a thumb-sized piece of peeled, crushed fresh ginger root and drink it as a tea.

GINGER AND TOFU STIR-FRY
serves 2

6 garlic cloves, crushed

2.5cm/1in piece root ginger, peeled and grated

cayenne pepper, to taste

200g/7oz firm tofu, diced

soy sauce, to cover

4 tbsp olive oil

1 broccoli head, cut into florets

1 green pepper, deseeded and chopped

400g/14oz bean sprouts

100g/3½oz/heaped 1 cup flaked almonds

Place the garlic, ginger, cayenne pepper and tofu in a bowl and drizzle over enough soy sauce to cover. Leave to marinate for 10 minutes. Heat the oil in a wok and add the tofu marinade, vegetables and bean sprouts, and stir-fry until lightly cooked. Add the almonds and stir through, then remove from the heat and serve.

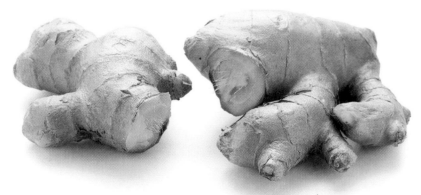

✦ GINGER AND LEMON DECOCTION
for sore throats

115g/4oz root ginger
500ml/17fl oz/2¼ cups water
juice and grated zest of 1 lemon
a pinch of cayenne pepper

Slice the ginger (there is no need to peel it) and put it in a pan with the water, lemon zest and cayenne pepper. Bring to the boil, reduce the heat and simmer, covered, for 20 minutes. Remove from the heat and add the lemon juice. Drink 1 cup according to symptoms. The decoction will keep for 2–3 days.

GINGER BEER

2l/70fl oz/8 cups bottled still mineral
    water
250g/9oz/1 cup sugar
¼ tsp dried yeast
juice of 1 lemon
1½–2 tbsp grated root ginger

Decant the water into another container. Pour the sugar into the empty bottle through a funnel, then add the yeast. Mix the lemon juice with the ginger, and pour into the bottle through the funnel. Add the water (leaving a 2.5cm/1in gap at the top). Shake well and leave in a warm place for 24–48 hours, then store in the fridge overnight. Pour into glasses through a strainer. Serve.

RASPBERRY AND GINGER WHIP

2 tsp grated root ginger
200g/7oz/1⅔ cups raspberries
450g/1lb crème fraiche
1 handful crystallized ginger, chopped

Put the root ginger and raspberries in a food processor and whizz. Add the mixture to the crème fraiche and stir. Serve chilled in individual dessert glasses, sprinkled with a few pieces of chopped crystallized ginger.

CREAMY GINGER DRESSING

4 tbsp tahini

2 tsp grated root ginger

1 garlic clove

1 tsp tamari

2 tsp brown rice syrup

Put all the ingredients in a blender with 5 tablespoons water and whizz until creamy. Serve stirred into noodles or as a salad dressing.

GINGERADE *serves 2*

1 tbsp caster sugar

55g/2oz root ginger, peeled
  and grated

250ml/9fl oz/1 cup sparkling
  mineral water

juice of ½ lemon

ice, to serve

Place the sugar, ginger and 250ml/ 9fl oz/1 cup water in a pan and bring to the boil. Reduce the heat, cover and simmer for 10 minutes. Leave to cool, then pass through a sieve. Stir into the sparkling mineral water, add the lemon juice and serve with ice.

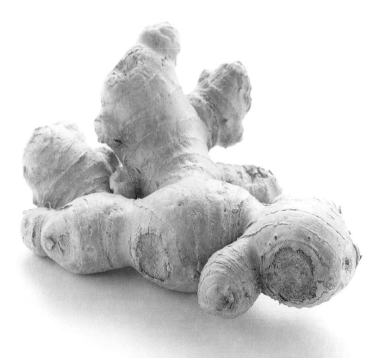

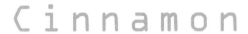

Cinnamon

VITAMINS B2, B3, B5, B6, E, K, BETA-CAROTENE, BIOTIN; CALCIUM, COPPER, IODINE, IRON, MAGNESIUM, MANGANESE, PHOSPHORUS, POTASSIUM, SELENIUM, ZINC; FIBRE

Highly prized since antiquity, cinnamon was regarded as a gift fit for kings and it is said that wars were even fought over it. With a long history of use in India, cinnamon is now one of the world's most important spices, with a plethora of healing properties.

Stimulating and warming, cinnamon is a traditional remedy for digestive problems, such as nausea, vomiting and diarrhoea, as well as for aching muscles and other symptoms of viral conditions such as colds and flu. Owing to its heating properties, it can promote sweating, thus helping to lower body temperature during fever. It can also be used for treating mild food poisoning, and is good for bleeding gums and as a mouthwash to counter halitosis.

Cinnamon has a surprisingly strong effect on the brain and moods, scientists have found. Its distinctive smell works directly on the brain to increase alertness. It has been found to help students concentrate more effectively in exams, and may slow down the onset of cognitive decline in old age. Research has shown that compounds in cinnamon stabilize blood-sugar levels, which in turn prevent mood swings and dips in blood sugar post-exercise – a time when even the most health-conscious athlete might be tempted to succumb to calorie-laden chocolate and sweets. As little as half a teaspoonful a day – sprinkled on porridge for breakfast or used to sweeten a cup of herbal tea – can make a difference and, say scientists, even help to control type-2 diabetes.

Cinnamon also has anti-bacterial and anti-fungal properties that have been found to inhibit organisms such as *Candida albicans*, a yeast responsible for causing candidiasis and thrush.

This powerful healing spice is also good for the heart and the circulatory system. Research has shown that it can significantly lower cholesterol levels. It also has a positive effect on blood platelets, preventing them from clumping together too much.

CINNAMON POACHED FRUIT

250ml/9fl oz/1 cup white wine
juice and grated zest of ½ lemon
2 tbsp ground cinnamon
4 pears, peeled, cored and chopped
8 apricots, pitted and chopped
4 tbsp chopped dried fruit of choice
yogurt, ricotta cheese or ice cream, to serve

Place the wine, lemon juice, zest and cinnamon into a large pan. Bring to the boil. Add the fruit and return to the boil. Reduce the heat and simmer for 2 minutes. Leave to stand for at least 10 minutes. Serve with yogurt, ricotta or ice cream.

CINNAMON CREAM

250g/9oz silken tofu
150ml/5fl oz/scant ⅔ cup apple juice
3 tbsp brown rice syrup
3 tbsp sunflower oil
½ tsp ground cinnamon

Put all the ingredients in a food processor and whizz until smooth and creamy. Use as a substitute for dairy cream on desserts.

APPLE AND CINNAMON PORRIDGE

2 cinnamon sticks
5 cloves
2 tsp sugar
2 apples, peeled and sliced
125g/4½oz/1¼ cups instant porridge oats

In a large pan, bring 750ml/26fl oz/ 3 cups water to the boil. Reduce the heat, add the cinnamon, cloves, sugar and apples, and simmer for 10 minutes. Remove the spices, stir in the oats and serve.

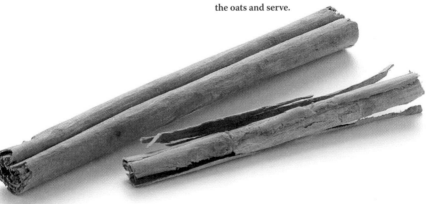

Green tea

Vitamins C, E, K; flavonoids; tannins

Not just a refreshingly different brew, green tea is also packed with powerful healing nutrients. This health-giving drink can help weight reduction while protecting against a wide range of diseases.

Tea is the most popular beverage in the world. It is grown in high areas in countries with warm, wet climates, such as Japan and India, but China is the biggest producer. Green tea comes from the same plant, *Camellia sinensis*, as ordinary black tea, but is processed differently, leaving important nutrients intact. Its leaves are lightly steamed when cut, rather than left to dry out like black tea. The medicinal properties of green tea have been recognized in the East for over 4,000 years and it is fast becoming recognized all over the world for its youth-enhancing properties. It has a fresh, astringent flavour.

Green tea is available both loose and in teabags, with added natural flavourings such as lemon and apple, and herbs such as digestion-soothing peppermint and brain-boosting ginkgo biloba to enhance the health benefits further. Choose high-quality gunpowder green tea if possible, preferably organic. Green tea is best drunk without milk, but you could add lemon or honey to taste.

Few foods excite scientists as much as green tea, with its phenomenal range of health benefits. This humble hot drink is a powerhouse of polyphenols – potent antioxidant flavonoids that neutralize damaging free radicals, helping to prevent diseases such as cancer and helping the body to stay youthful. Tea's polyphenols include catechins, which counteract cancer-causing agents. It is also anti-inflammatory and can prevent flare-ups of allergic conditions such as asthma. Its anti-bacterial abilities mean it can fight tooth decay and gum disease.

Green tea plays a dual role in helping you to shape up: firstly by increasing exercise endurance and secondly by inhibiting the action of enzymes that help to turn food into fat, especially around the midriff, where stored fat increases the risk of heart disease and diabetes.

This wonderdrink contains phenolic compounds that help to strengthen blood vessels, which makes it excellent for treating conditions such as thread or varicose veins, as well as cold hands or feet. It also contains good amounts of vitamin E to help to boost immunity, promote healthy, glowing skin and protect the eyes and the heart. The tannins in green tea offer further benefits for the eyes, as they act as an anti-inflammatory to relieve puffiness.

Green tea can help to lower blood pressure and cholesterol and stop the hardening of the arteries, reducing the risk of heart disease and strokes. The antioxidant flavonoids in green tea offer fantastic protection against heart and circulatory problems and have anti-carcinogenic properties. They lower "bad" LDL cholesterol and triglyceride levels and raise "good" HDL cholesterol levels. They also help to ward off wrinkles and preserve eye health.

You can enjoy the benefits of green tea by drinking 3 to 4 cups a day. Use boiling water to gain the full health benefits, or slightly cooler water if you prefer a less bitter taste. To take advantage of all its nutrients, you need to brew it for five minutes and drink it strong. However, some people find this too bitter and compromise by drinking it weaker.

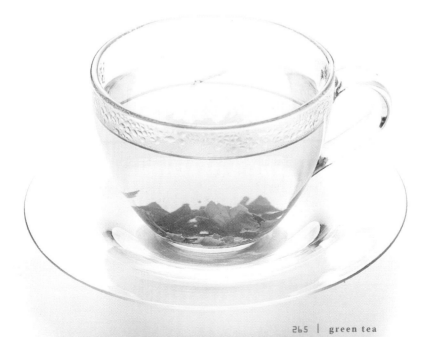

GREEN TEA AND PEACH REFRESHER

2 peaches, stoned and sliced
1.5l/52fl oz/6 cups cold water
6 green tea teabags
clear honey, to taste
mint sprigs, to serve

Put the peaches in a pan, add the water and bring to the boil. Put the teabags in a large pitcher and pour the water and peaches over them. Steep for 6 minutes, remove the bags and add the honey to taste. Allow to cool, then refrigerate until chilled. Pour the tea and peach slices into glasses and garnish with mint to serve.

MORROCAN MINT TEA

2 tbsp gunpowder green tea
1 litre/35fl oz/4 cups boiling water
1 large bunch fresh mint
brown sugar, to taste (optional)

Place the tea in a teapot, cover with boiling water and leave to steep for 3 minutes. Pull out a few mint sprigs to save for each serving, then add the rest to the pot and leave for a further 5 minutes. Pour into glasses, adding sugar if desired, and decorate with the saved mint sprigs.

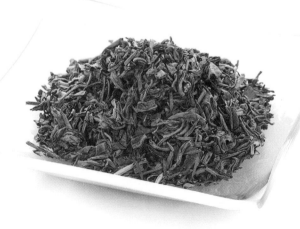

Chamomile

FLAVONOIDS, TANNINS, COUMARINS, VALERIANIC ACID

Best known as a relaxant, this medicinal plant is one of the most widely used healing herbs and is a popular remedy for insomnia and digestive complaints.

There are two main species of chamomile, which are known as Roman and German chamomile. While both have great therapeutic properties, German chamomile is more widely available.

Usually made into a tea, chamomile relaxes the muscles throughout the body. Its bitters stimulate the flow of bile and the secretion of digestive juices, enhancing the appetite and improving sluggish digestion. The herb has sedative properties and is very soothing, helping to induce relaxation and sleep.

Chamomile contains antioxidant flavonoids, which help to fight harmful free radicals and protect against infection. One of these flavonoids, quercetin, also has powerful anti-inflammatory properties.

Used topically, chamomile treats inflamed joints and stiff muscles. It also has cosmetic benefits – when used in face creams, it promotes a youthful, glowing complexion. Chamomile is also known for being a powerful conditioner that leaves the hair softer and shinier.

---

*CHAMOMILE TREATMENT
to condition the hair throats

1 handful chamomile flowers
80ml/2½fl oz/⅓ cup olive oil

Combine the chamomile and oil in a jar with a lid. Stand on a sunny windowsill and shake at least once a day. After 2 weeks, strain and discard the chamomile. Apply to the ends of your hair, avoiding the scalp, using about 2–4 teaspoonfuls, depending on hair length. Leave on for 10 minutes, then shampoo as normal.

Honey

VITAMINS B2, B3, B5, B6, BIOTIN, FOLIC ACID; CALCIUM, COPPER, IRON, MAGNESIUM, MANGANESE, PHOSPHORUS, POTASSIUM, SELENIUM, SODIUM, ZINC; CAFFEIC ACID, PROPOLIS; CARBOHYDRATE

Ancient societies around the world used honey as an energy food. It has evolved as a unique and powerful remedy for a wide variety of complaints.

So prized was the food of bees that the Romans used it instead of gold to pay their taxes. Today, honey has become known as "liquid gold" because of its outstanding nutritive and healing properties.

Composed of 38 per cent fructose, 31 per cent glucose, 1 per cent sucrose and 9 per cent other sugars, honey is the only natural sweetener that requires no additional refining or processing. The rest comprises water and small amounts of vitamins, including vitamin B6, which is good for the brain, and many minerals, including calcium and magnesium to strengthen the bones and selenium and zinc to support the immune system. It helps with any tendency towards hypoglycaemia, which may contribute towards insomnia and mood swings. It also provides many nutritional substances, including vitamins B2 and B3, necessary for thyroid function, and pantothenic acid (vitamin B5), which plays an important role in energy production. Honey is also rich in trace amounts of essential minerals such as copper, iron, manganese, phosphorus, potassium and sodium.

A recognized antioxidant, honey is a powerful, broad-spectrum antibiotic with both anti-fungal and anti-microbial properties, acting against organisms that encourage *Staphylococcus* bacteria as well as candida fungal infections. Honey also contains an amazing substance called propolis, which helps to prevent and treat coughs and colds, as well as stomach disorders – recent research suggests that it can counteract food-poisoning bacteria.

The extraordinary antibacterial content found in the Manuka honey of New Zealand has been shown to inhibit the growth of many bacteria, including *Helicobacter pylori*, which is associated with causing most stomach and duodenal ulcers. The antibacterial activity of this honey is also proving to be an effective weapon in combating superbugs such as MRSA (Methicillin-resistant *Staphylococcus aureus*), strains of which have become particularly resistant to conventional antibiotic treatment. Moreover, because it also has potent anti-fungal properties, this special honey has been used effectively to treat athlete's foot and other fungal infections. Unfiltered honey contains pollen grains and helps hayfever.

Honey also contains phytonutrients such as caffeic acid, which has anti-carcinogenic properties. As an energy source, it enhances sports performance by providing a welcome boost both during and after exercise. No wonder honey is considered a general pick-me-up!

Used topically, honey has a powerful antiseptic effect for the treatment of ulcers, burns and wounds. It has an anti-inflammatory action, reducing swelling and pain, and by stimulating the regrowth of tissue under the skin's surface, honey helps the healing mechanism. It is also a humectant, attracting and retaining water, which keeps the skin soft and supple. This makes it a popular ingredient in beauty creams.

HONEY CITRUS JUICE

2 grapefruit, peeled and broken into
   segments
3 lemons, peeled and quartered
4cm/1½in piece root ginger, peeled and
   cut into chunks
1 tbsp clear honey

Press alternate chunks of grapefruit, lemon and ginger through a juicer. Add the honey, stir well and drink immediately.

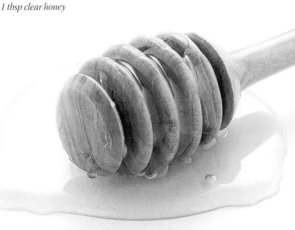

✦HONEY DRESSING *for wounds*

honey
gauze bandage

Spread some honey onto a gauze bandage and apply it to the wound. The amount of honey used depends on the amount of fluid exuding from the wound. Large amounts of exudate require substantial amounts of honey. Reapply the dressing as necessary.

HONEY ALMOND CUP

500ml/17fl oz/2 cups rice milk
200g/7oz/1⅓ cups blanched almonds
2 tbsp clear honey
1 tbsp natural vanilla extract

Put the rice milk and almonds in a blender with 300ml/10½fl oz/1¼ cups water and mix well. Pour the liquid through a sieve into a glass pitcher. Stir in the honey and vanilla extract, then chill in the fridge. Serve.

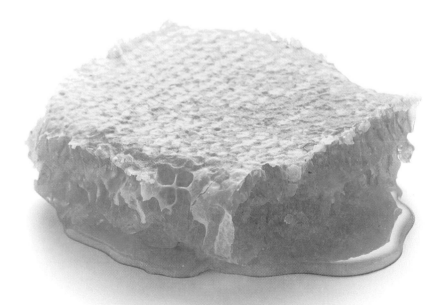

*HONEY FACE MASK
to firm the skin

1 tbsp clear honey

1 egg white

1 tsp glycerin

30g/1oz/¼ cup plain flour

In a small bowl, mix the honey, egg white and glycerin. Then, add enough of the flour to form a paste. Smooth the mask over the face and throat. Leave for 10 minutes, then rinse off.

HONEY VINAIGRETTE

2 tbsp clear honey

2 tbsp cider vinegar

3 tbsp extra virgin olive oil

1 tsp French mustard (optional)

a pinch of of salt

Pour the honey and cider vinegar into a pan and place over a low heat until just warm. Gently add the olive oil, beating the mixture with a fork. Remove from the heat, then add the mustard, if using, and the salt. Serve with a warm salad, such as chicken.

BANANA, HONEY AND PEANUT BAGELS

4 wholegrain bagels

6 tbsp crunchy peanut butter

4 bananas

4 tsp clear honey

½ tsp ground cinnamon

Carefully cut the bagels in half and spread each side with peanut butter. Set aside. In a bowl, chop and mash the bananas and mix them with the honey and cinnamon. Spoon the mixture on top of the peanut butter. Grill the bagel halves for a few minutes, topping side up, and serve immediately.

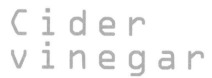

Cider vinegar

VITAMINS B1, B2, B6, C, E, BETA-CAROTENE; CALCIUM, CHLORINE, FLUORINE, IRON, MAGNESIUM, MANGANESE, PHOSPHORUS, POTASSIUM, SELENIUM, SODIUM, SILICA, SULPHUR, ZINC; MALIC ACID, ASCETIC ACID; PECTIN; FIBRE

Made from fermented apple juice and rich in enzymes, cider vinegar has been used for centuries to aid digestion. It is thought that Hippocrates, the father of modern medicine, used apple cider vinegar as a healing elixir to treat his patients.

More than ninety different beneficial substances have been discovered in cider vinegar, including carbolic acids, enzymes and trace minerals, which help to balance the body's acid–alkaline levels. Through its alkalizing effect, it is reported to alleviate a number of complaints, such as rheumatism, headaches, heartburn and muscle cramps.

The malic acid content of cider vinegar helps to dissolve calcium deposits in the body and eases arthritis. It also helps to balance the body's acid–alkaline pH levels and oxygenates the blood, thus aiding digestion and boosting the immune system. Enzyme-rich, cider vinegar contains a perfect balance of minerals, as well as apple pectin, the water-soluble dietary fibre that binds to toxins in the body and assists in their removal, thus improving the elimination of waste. Pectin also lowers cholesterol levels, and so helps to stave off heart disease.

Taking a few drops of cider vinegar with or before a meal has been proved to help people lose weight. It has the added benefit of reducing the indigestion that can accompany a change in diet, which can cause pangs that feel like hunger even when you've just eaten. Vinegar's acetic acid content makes you feel full up sooner and for longer. This feeling of satiety stems from a reduction in the glycaemic index (GI) of the food you eat. Foods with a high GI (including most highly processed items) go through your system quickly, leaving you ready for more. Vinegar reduces the GI and lets food stay longer in your stomach. It also reduces the risk of a mid-afternoon energy slump sending you in search of a snack.

✦ OXYMEL *for respiratory ailments*

cider vinegar
clear honey
water

Combine equal amounts of apple cider vinegar and honey in a glass jar. Shake to combine. Take 1 teaspoon when you have specific symptoms, or add eight times the amount of water to create a juice for regular sipping.

✳ CIDER VINEGAR HAIR RINSE
to restore dull, lifeless hair

2 tbsp cider vinegar
750ml/26fl oz/3 cups water

Mix the cider vinegar and water in a jug. After shampooing and conditioning your hair as usual, pour the cider vinegar mixture over your hair as a final rinse.

CREAMY SALAD DRESSING

2 tbsp cider vinegar
2 tsp apple juice
4 tbsp plain bio-yogurt
1 garlic clove, crushed
1 tsp chopped thyme

Place all the ingredients in a bowl and whisk together. Chill and serve the dressing on your favourite salad.

Tofu

Vitamins A, K; calcium, copper, iron, magnesium, manganese, phosphorus, potassium, selenium; omega-3 and -6 essential fatty acids; fibre; protein; tryptophan; isoflavones

One of the best vegetarian forms of protein, tofu works well in everything from smoothies to stir-fries. This wonder-working soya product can protect your organs while also helping you to lose weight.

Made fom the curds of soya milk, which gives it its alternative name "bean curd", tofu is a versatile, low-fat food jam-packed with nutrients. It is available in traditional Chinese block form or in the smoother Japanese silken form. Both come in a range of textures from soft to extra-firm. Soft tofu blends easily in smoothies and desserts, while firm tofu works well in main meals.

While it is perhaps best known for its beneficial effects on women's hormones, tofu may also help both sexes to maintain a healthy weight. Among soya's many healthy components is an isoflavone that seems to promote fat loss by reducing the size and number of fat cells. Women using tofu to treat menopausal symptoms have found that it also prevented weight gain, especially on the abdomen, which is an area commonly affected by the changes in the body's reproductive hormone levels after the menstrual cycle stops.

Research has shown that people who regularly eat tofu can lower their "bad" (LDL) cholesterol levels by as much as a third, making it a powerful protector of the heart and cardiovascular system. Tofu is also a good source of omega-3 fatty acids and fibre, which both support heart health as well as helping to stave off food cravings. Like all soya products, tofu is rich in calcium and magnesium to build strong bones.

Although tofu has been shown to reduce the risk of many serious diseases, including cancers, heart disease, osteoporosis and diabetes, its powerful effects on hormones can also stimulate hormone-dependent cancers or thyroid problems, so it should not be overused. Traditional tofu is the healthiest option – the long-term effects of new products are not known and so it is best to avoid them.

TOFU SKEWERS

4 tbsp soy sauce
1 tbsp sesame oil
1 tbsp apple juice
a pinch of chilli powder
450g/1lb firm tofu, drained and cubed
4 sweet peppers, deseeded and chopped
  into chunks

Mix together the soy sauce, sesame oil, apple juice and chilli powder and marinate the tofu for 1 hour. Thread the tofu and peppers alternately onto skewers. Grill or bake for 5–10 minutes until brown, basting often with the remaining marinade. Serve.

TOFU SMOOTHIE

200g/7oz tofu
125ml/4fl oz/½ cup orange juice
125ml/4fl oz/½ cup mango pulp
4 apples, cored and chopped
4 tbsp chopped walnuts

Put all the ingredients except for 1 tablespoon of the walnuts in a blender. Whizz on a low speed until the ingredients are mixed, then on a high speed until the mixture is smooth. Pour into glasses, top with the remaining walnuts, and serve.

BLUEBERRY AND TOFU MOUSSE

200g/7oz silken tofu
250g/9oz/1⅔ cups blueberries
85g/3oz/¾ cup ground almonds
1 tsp ground cinnamon
1 tsp lemon juice
2 tsp toasted, flaked almonds

Whizz the tofu and blueberries in a food processor. Add the ground almonds, cinnamon and lemon juice. Spoon the mousse into four bowls and sprinkle over the almond flakes.

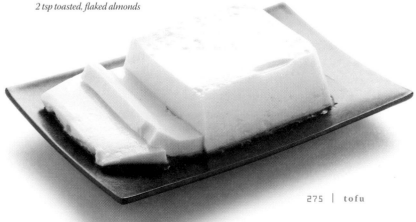

Ailments directory

ANAEMIA

This condition occurs when there is a decrease in the amount of oxygen-carrying haemoglobin in our red blood cells. The first sign is usually weakness or exhaustion. Symptoms include feeling tired all the time, pale skin, breathlessness and pale inner lower eyelids. The likeliest cause is lack of iron or vitamin B12. Young women, in particular, are at risk, especially if they have heavy periods and eat little or no meat, as the body absorbs iron more easily from meat or fish than from any other source. Foods rich in vitamin C help the body to absorb iron. If the exhaustion continues, see your doctor.

Foods to eat: apple (p.26); pineapple (p.36); papaya (p.42); strawberry (p.52); plum (p.56); apricot (p.58); asparagus (p.78); globe artichoke (p.80); beetroot (p.82); sweet potato (p.90); broccoli (p.94); spinach (p.100); cabbage (p.104); fennel (p.124); alfalfa (p.130); watercress (p.132); seaweed (p.134); lamb (p.142); beef (p.144); turkey (p.146); bio-yogurt (p.151); milk (p.154); egg (p.156); salmon (p.164); oyster (p.172); flaxseed (p.192); quinoa (p.214); millet (p.221); rye (p.222); chickpea (p.232); lentil (p.234); chilli (p.252); cayenne pepper (p.254); turmeric (p.256); cider vinegar (p.272)

ARTHRITIS

Osteoarthritis is caused by wear and tear on the joints, so most people have at least a few twinges by the time they reach their 50s. It may also happen earlier at the site of an injury. The degenerative disease rheumatoid arthritis is much less common but often starts in younger people. They're different conditions, but both may respond to the anti-inflammatory effects of foods rich in omega-3, especially oily fish (though oily fish is not recommended for anyone with the form of arthritis called gout). Calcium, iron and vitamin D have shown some good effects on arthritis. A diet rich in fruit and vegetables provides many other phytonutrients that are believed to be helpful.

Foods to eat: pineapple (p.36); papaya (p.42); cherry (p.48); raspberry (p.54); pomegranate (p.60); olive and olive oil (p.72); beetroot (p.82); broccoli (p.94); cabbage (p.104); onion (p.108); celery (p.110); squash (p.116); aubergine (p.118); mushroom (p.120); seaweed (p.134); salmon (p.164); walnut (p.178); sesame seed and oil (p.196); oats (p.210); parsley (p.240); turmeric (p.256); ginger (p.258); cider vinegar (p.272)

ASTHMA AND LUNG DISEASE

Asthma sufferers experience inflamed air passages of the lungs. This can cause extra-sensitivity to "triggers" or allergens, including milk, wheat, nuts and fish, which may be best avoided.

Foods rich in vitamin C have long been known to fight asthma and other chest diseases. Other nutrients are now known to help in different ways: magnesium, for example, helps to prevent the breath-restricting spasms of an asthma attack.

Foods to eat: *orange (p.18); kiwi fruit (p.38); papaya (p.42); raspberry (p.54); olive and olive oil (p.72); carrot (p.86); sweet potato (p.90); broccoli (p.94); kale (p.98); onion (p.108); pepper (p.112); squash (p.116); mushroom (p.120); fennel (p.124); seaweed (p.134); salmon (p.164); walnut (p.178); flaxseed (p.192); peppermint (p.244); rosemary (p.246); garlic (p.248); cayenne pepper (p.254); green tea (p.264)*

CANCER

Healthy eating could prevent up to a third of all cancers, according to the World Health Organization. There are a huge number of naturally occurring phytonutrients shown to reduce cancer risk. Fruits and vegetables of every kind offer slightly different beneficial compounds.

Foods to eat: *lemon (p.14); orange (p.18); grapefruit (p.20); apple (p.26); pear (p.30); grape (p.34); blueberry (p.44); cherry (p.48); cranberry (p.50); strawberry (p.52); raspberry (p.54); prune (p.56); pomegranate (p.60); Cantaloupe melon (p.62); tomato (p.68); olive and olive oil (p.72); asparagus (p.78); globe artichoke (p.80); beetroot (p.82); carrot (p.86); potato (p.88); sweet potato (p.90); yam (p.92); broccoli (p.94); kale (p.98); spinach (p.100); Brussels sprout (p.102); cabbage (p.104); cauliflower (p.106); onion (p.108); celery (p.110); pepper (p.112); squash (p.116); aubergine (p.118); mushroom (p.120); fennel (p.124); lettuce (p.126); cucumber (p.128); alfalfa (p.130); watercress (p.132); seaweed (p.134); beef (p.144); turkey (p.146); bio-yogurt (p.151); salmon (p.164); prawn (p.170); walnut (p.178); almond (p.182); Brazil nut (p.188); flaxseed (p.192); oats (p.210); brown rice (p.216); rye (p.222); chickpea (p.232); garlic (p.248); turmeric (p.256); ginger (p.258); green tea (p.264)*

COMMON COLD AND FLU

Flu is a viral infection with extreme cold-like symptoms. Avoiding dairy products and eating fruits and vegetables can help to fight both types of virus. Use foods and herbs that help to boost immunity.

Foods to eat: *lemon (p.14); orange (p.18); grapefruit (p.20); blueberry (p.44); cranberry (p.50); raspberry (p.54); pomegranate (p.60); tomato (p.68); carrot (p.86); potato (p.88); sweet potato (p.90); broccoli (p.94); onion (p.108); pepper (p.112); mushroom (p.120); lettuce (p.126); watercress (p.132); seaweed (p.134); prawn (p.170); oats (p.210); sage (p.242); peppermint (p.244); rosemary (p.246); garlic (p.248); chilli (p.252); ginger (p.258); cinnamon (p.262); honey (p.268)*

COUGHS AND BRONCHITIS

If you have a cough or bronchitis – an infection of the bronchial tube lining – it is best to avoid dairy products, which are mucus-creating.

Foods to eat: *lemon (p.14); orange (p.18); apricot (p.58); carrot (p.86); sweet potato (p.90); onion (p.108); watercress (p.132); flaxseed (p.192); sunflower seed and oil (p.198); aduki bean (p.228); sage (p.242); rosemary (p.246); garlic (p.248); chilli (p.252); ginger (p.258); honey (p.268)*

CYSTITIS

Urinary tract infections, such as cystitis, cause pain and difficulty in passing urine. They must always be treated promptly, as they can spread fast and affect the kidneys. Vitamin C combats infection, and some foods discourage bacteria from sticking to the bladder wall. These foods are a back-up to medical treatment, and they reduce the risk of recurrence.

Foods to eat: *blueberry (p.44); cherry (p.48); cranberry (p.50); raspberry (p.54); asparagus (p.78); Brussels sprout (p.102); celery (p.110); fennel (p.124); alfalfa (p.130); bio-yogurt (p.151); sesame seed and oil (p.196); barley (p.208); quinoa (p.214); aduki bean (p.228); chickpea (p.232); garlic (p.248)*

DEPRESSION (MILD)

Characterized by tearfulness, anxiety and feelings of hopelessness, mild depression is a condition experienced by one in four people at some stage in their lives. Cutting out alcohol, cigarettes and sugary foods, and eating those high in omega-3 fatty acids and B-vitamins is thought to help. Exercise is also known to increase the feel-good factor. The body converts nutrients into message-carrying chemicals that have a direct effect on our emotions. Cheer yourself up with foods rich in tryptophan, selenium, B-vitamins and protein.

Foods to eat: banana (p.23); raspberry (p.54); apricot (p.58); avocado (p.64); sweet potato (p.90); spinach (p.100); seaweed (p.134); milk (p.154); egg (p.156); tuna (p.162); salmon (p.164); oyster (p.172); walnut (p.178); almond (p.182); Brazil nut (p.188); flaxseed (p.192); sunflower seed and oil (p.198); oats (p.210); quinoa (p.214); brown rice (p.216); buckwheat (p.220)

DIABETES

Diabetes is a disease in which the body either fails to produce enough insulin or doesn't respond properly to the insulin produced. Foods that release glucose slowly into the bloodstream help to keep diabetes under control, and may also reduce the risk of developing this condition. Avoid processed foods and, although dried fruit and juices are healthy foods, limit these as they are rich in sugars.

Foods to eat: orange (p.18); grapefruit (p.20); apple (p.26); blueberry (p.44); avocado (p.64); globe artichoke (p.80); carrot (p.86); sweet potato (p.90); yam (p.92); mushroom (p.120); seaweed (p.134); turkey (p.146); walnut (p.178); almond (p.182); barley (p.208); oats (p.210); quinoa (p.214); brown rice (p.216); buckwheat (p.220); millet (p.221); chickpea (p.232); lentil (p.234); garlic (p.248); cinnamon (p.262); green tea (p.264); tofu (p.274)

DIGESTIVE COMPLAINTS see also Irritable Bowel Syndrome, p.282

The key to keeping the digestive system in good shape is to eat plenty of fibre-rich foods and drink lots of water. If you suffer from indigestion – discomfort, or a burning feeling in the oesophagus – try to reduce your intake of acid-forming foods, such as cheese and red meat, and eat more foods containing digestive enzymes and fibre.

Foods to eat: grapefruit (p.20); banana (p.23); grape (p.34); papaya (p.42); globe artichoke (p.80); carrot (p.86); Brussels sprout (p.102); fennel (p.124); watercress (p.132); bio-yogurt (p.151); almond (p.182); coconut and coconut oil (p.190); wheat and wheatgerm (p.206); barley (p.208); brown rice (p.216); buckwheat (p.220); millet (p.221); chickpea (p.232); peppermint (p.244); garlic (p.248); cayenne pepper (p.254); ginger (p.258); cinnamon (p.262); chamomile (p.267); cider vinegar (p.272)

ECZEMA

Eczema describes a group of inflammatory skin conditions that make the skin itchy, irritated and red, sometimes with blisters. There are a number of causes, ranging from household cleaning products to certain foods to stress. In order to manage the condition it is important to identify and avoid any common allergens. A diet rich in essential fatty acids, vitamin A and zinc can help.

Foods to eat: papaya (p.42); avocado (p.64); tomato (p.68); olive and olive oil (p.72); carrot (p.86); cucumber (p.128); seaweed (p.134); salmon (p.164); walnut (p.178); pine nut (p.181); flaxseed (p.192); sunflower seed and oil (p.198); pumpkin seed (p.200); oats (p.210); quinoa (p.214); rosemary (p.246); cayenne pepper (p.254); turmeric (p.256); chamomile (p.267)

EYE DISEASE

If you want to keep your eyes shiny and bright, remember the old adage about eating your carrots – or, in fact, any brightly coloured fruit and vegetables. Studies suggest that the antioxidants they contain – including vitamins A, C and E, and lutein – benefit the eyes by helping the lenses to adjust to changes in light; maintaining the macula (the part of the eye that enables clear vision); and keeping the eyes moist.

Foods to eat: kiwi fruit (p.38); blueberry (p.44); cherry (p.48); apricot (p.58); pomegranate (p.60); asparagus (p.78); beetroot (p.82); carrot (p.86); broccoli (p.94); kale (p.98); spinach (p.100); pepper (p.112); watercress (p.132); seaweed (p.134); lamb (p.142); bio-yogurt (p.151); egg (p.156); sesame seed and oil (p.196); pumpkin seed (p.200); barley (p.208)

FATIGUE *see also Post-viral Fatigue, p.284*

If you're getting seven to eight hours' sleep a night but feel exhausted most of the time, you may not be eating all the many nutrients you need, including protein, B-vitamins and an array of minerals. This often happens when you're busy, too, and living on fast food.

Unexplained fatigue can be a sign of something more serious, such as Post-viral Fatigue, so if cutting down on stress, working sensible hours and eating well doesn't help, seek medical advice.

Foods to eat: orange (p.18); banana (p.23); raspberry (p.54); prune (p.56); avocado (p.64); asparagus (p.78); globe artichoke (p.80); potato (p.88); sweet potato (p.90); yam (p.92); spinach (p.100); celery (p.110); squash (p.116); mushroom (p.120); cucumber (p.128); lamb (p.142); beef (p.144); tuna (p.162); sardine (p.168); oyster (p.172); almond (p.182); cashew nut (p.186); Brazil nut (p.188); coconut and coconut oil (p.190); sunflower seed and oil (p.198); pumpkin seed (p.200); barley (p.208); oats (p.210); quinoa (p.214); brown rice (p.216); millet (p.221); soya bean (p.224); kidney bean (p.230); chickpea (p.232); lentil (p.234); rosemary (p.246); honey (p.268)

HEADACHES AND MIGRAINE

These can be triggered by many different stimuli, from fatigue to expansion of blood vessels in the head. They may be prevented, or relieved, by foods rich in omega-3 fats, vitamin B2, magnesium or calcium. Some migraines can be triggered by eating preserved meat, strong cheeses, pickles, fatty foods, coffee or the artificial sweetener aspartame.

Foods to eat: *seaweed (p.134); milk (p.154); rye (p.222); chickpea (p.232); peppermint (p.244); rosemary (p.246); cayenne pepper (p.254)*

HEART DISEASE

One of the main causes of heart disease is the blockage of arteries by cholesterol. Following an exercise regime and eating monounsaturated fats (found in olive oil, nuts, seeds and fish) instead of saturated fats (found in animal products and processed foods) can make a dramatic difference to your heart health.

Healthy eating is proven to play a major role in preventing or alleviating heart disease. All kinds of fruit and vegetables are especially valuable because of their flavonoids and fibre content, particularly when they are replacing high-fat foods or heavily processed items that are low in nutritional value.

Foods to eat: *grapefruit (p.20); apple (p.26); pear (p.30); grape (p.34); kiwi fruit (p.38); papaya (p.42); blueberry (p.44); cherry (p.48); cranberry (p.50); raspberry (p.54); apricot (p.58); pomegranate (p.60); Cantaloupe melon (p.62); avocado (p.64); tomato (p.68); olive and olive oil (p.72); asparagus (p.78); globe artichoke (p.80); carrot (p.86); broccoli (p.94); spinach (p.100); cabbage (p.104); onion (p.108); celery (p.110); pepper (p.112); squash (p.116); aubergine (p.118); mushroom (p.120); fennel (p.124); watercress (p.132); seaweed (p.134); tuna (p.162); salmon (p.164); sardine (p.168); oyster (p.172); walnut (p.178); almond (p.182);*

cashew nut (p.186); coconut and coconut oil (p.190); flaxseed (p.192); sesame seed and oil (p.196); sunflower seed and oil (p.198); pumpkin seed (p.200); barley (p.208); oats (p.210); quinoa (p.214); brown rice (p.216); buckwheat (p.220); millet (p.221); soya bean (p.224); chickpea (p.232); lentil (p.234); garlic (p.248); turmeric (p.256); ginger (p.258); green tea (p.264); tofu (p.274)

HIGH BLOOD PRESSURE

Hypertension, or high blood pressure, means that the heart has to work harder to pump blood around the body, and increases the risk of heart disease and strokes. You can bring it down through exercise, stress reduction and losing excess weight.

It also helps if you avoid high-fat and salt-laden dishes and opt instead for foods loaded with magnesium, vitamin C, essential fatty acids and fibre, such as fruit and vegetables.

Foods to eat: orange (p.18); banana (p.23); apple (p.26); fig (p.32); grape (p.34); pomegranate (p.60); avocado (p.64); olive and olive oil (p.72); potato (p.88); broccoli (p.94); spinach (p.100); celery (p.110); mushroom (p.120); seaweed (p.134); salmon (p.164); flaxseed (p.192); sesame seed and oil (p.196); oats (p.210); buckwheat (p.220); lentil (p.234); parsley (p.240); garlic (p.248)

IRRITABLE BOWEL SYNDROME (IBS)

This distressing and sometimes painful condition can involve consti-pation, diarrhoea, flatulence, nausea or all of these afflictions. Bouts of irritable bowel syndrome may be triggered by stress or by certain foods, such as dairy products, gluten, spicy foods or the artificial sweetener sorbitol. Tea, coffee and alcohol can also have an irritating effect.

As irritable bowel syndrome sometimes develops from chronic constipation, it may be relieved by the same remedies: exercise every day, plenty of fluids, regular meals not too late in the evening and unhurried bowel movements. If flatulence is a problem, avoid eating a lot of pulses.

Foods to eat: apple (p.26); pear (p.30); fig (p.32); raspberry (p.54); prune (p.56); asparagus (p.78); globe artichoke (p.80); fennel (p.124); cucumber (p.128); bio-yogurt (p.151); flaxseed (p.192); oats (p.210); brown rice (p.216); millet (p.221); peppermint (p.244); rosemary (p.246); ginger (p.258); chamomile (p.267)

JOINT PROBLEMS

Regular exercise can place a strain on the joints. For example, knee pain is a common running injury. It's possible to protect joints from injury and wear and tear by maintaining the correct weight for your height and by alternating periods of heavy activity with periods of rest to avoid repetitive stress on your joints. Research also shows that eating foods rich in essential fatty acids can help to protect the cartilage cells that facilitate joint movement.

Keep your joints supple by eating antioxidant-rich fruits and vegetables, along with nuts, seeds and oily fish. Some spices, such as cayenne pepper, may be used topically to help to relieve aching joints.

Foods to eat: *apple (p.26); pineapple (p.36); cherry (p.48); avocado (p.64); olive oil and olive (p.72); fennel (p.124); salmon (p.164); oyster (p.172); walnut (p.178); flaxseed (p.192); sesame seed and oil (p.196); sunflower seed and oil (p.198); wheat and wheatgerm (p.206); lentil (p.234); parsley (p.240); garlic (p.248); cayenne pepper (p.254); turmeric (p.256); ginger (p.258); chamomile (p.267); cider vinegar (p.272)*

MEMORY LOSS

As we get older, our bodies start to make fewer of the chemicals our brain cells need to work, thus making it harder to recall information. Studies have shown that vitamin E, magnesium and other nutrients may help to counteract this and so prevent memory loss. Researchers are also studying the possibility that foods rich in antioxidants, – particularly vitamins C and E and silica – might help to keep our brains active in later life.

Forgetfulness, inability to concentrate and "brain fog" can stem from many causes, often including stress and tiredness. Some nutrients are known to help keep your brain sharp at any age, including omega-3 oils and compounds in certain herbs. These may also delay or prevent mental deterioration in later life.

Foods to eat: *fig (p.32); mango (p.40); blueberry (p.44); olive and olive oil (p.72); beetroot (p.82); kale (p.98); spinach (p.100); cabbage (p.104); pepper (p.112); watercress (p.132); seaweed (p.134); milk (p.154); egg (p.156); salmon (p.164); prawn (p.170); oyster (p.172); walnut (p.178); flaxseed (p.192); sunflower seed and oil (p.198); pumpkin seed (p.200); wheat and wheatgerm (p.206); millet (p.221); kidney bean (p.230); parsley (p.240); sage (p.242); rosemary (p.246); cayenne pepper (p.254); turmeric (p.256); cinnamon (p.262); green tea (p.264)*

MENOPAUSAL SYMPTOMS

Levels of the reproductive hormone oestrogen can rise and fall sharply during the few years leading up to the menopause, and then decline steeply afterwards. This sometimes causes disruptive symptoms, which can be alleviated through healthy eating.

Phytoestrogens help to replace some of the missing oestrogen. Foods rich in vitamin E can reduce the severity of hot flushes and prevent night sweats causing insomnia. Depression, fatigue and memory loss may also occur during this time.

Foods to eat: olive and olive oil (p.72); alfalfa (p.130); seaweed (p.134); flaxseed (p.192); sunflower seed and oil (p.198); brown rice (p.216); rye (p.222); soya bean (p.224); sage (p.242); tofu (p.274)

OSTEOPOROSIS

Osteoporosis causes bones to become weak and brittle, so that you are more prone to fractures and breaks. Eating foods rich in calcium, as well as phosphorus and magnesium, can help to prevent the disease. Making sure you spend plenty of time outside also helps, as the sun triggers the production of vitamin D in the body, which helps to turn the calcium you eat into bone.

Building strong bones before you reach your 30s reduces the risk that you'll suffer from this condition in later life. Weight-bearing exercise is another vital way in which to protect bone health for the future.

Dairy foods and oily fish also provide vitamin D. Vitamin K and several other minerals are also important. All of these can also delay the progression of osteoporosis if you already have it.

Foods to eat: fig (p.32); pineapple (p.36); cherry (p.48); olive and olive oil (p.72); broccoli (p.94); kale (p.98); spinach (p.100); onion (p.108); lettuce (p.126); cucumber (p.128); watercress (p.132); seaweed (p.134); beef (p.144); chicken (p.148); bio-yogurt (p.151); milk (p.154); sardine (p.168); prawn (p.170); oyster (p.172); cashew nut (p.186); flaxseed (p.192); sesame seed and oil (p.196); pumpkin seed (p.200); oats (p.210); quinoa (p.214); millet (p.221); rye (p.222); soya bean (p.224); parsley (p.240); cayenne pepper (p.254); ginger (p.258); tofu (p.274)

POST-VIRAL FATIGUE (ME)

Although the specific cause of post-viral fatigue is still unknown, it often follows on from a viral illness and is more likely to occur in athletes who over-train. This chronic condition is characterized by low energy levels, fatigue and poor concentration. Eating plenty of immunity-boosting fruit and vegetables can help to alleviate the symptoms.

Foods to eat: grape (p.34); cherry (p.48); apricot (p.58); beetroot (p.82); carrot (p.86); pepper (p.112); peppermint (p.244); garlic (p.248)

PREMENSTRUAL SYNDROME (PMS)
If you feel depressed or irritable during the couple of days before a period, but fine once it starts, you probably suffer from premenstrual syndrome. Although you may be tempted to reach for sugary or fatty comfort foods, these can make the symptoms worse. However, foods rich in vitamins B6, D and E, and magnesium and calcium can help a lot.

Foods to eat: banana (p.23); sweet potato (p.90); seaweed (p.134); chicken (p.148); milk (p.154); oyster (p.172); flaxseed (p.192); millet (p.221); rosemary (p.246); turmeric (p.256); chamomile (p.267)

STOMACH ULCERS
These painful patches of damage to the stomach wall are now acknowleged to be caused by the bacterium *Helicobacter pylori*, and can often be cured by antibiotics. Stomach ulcers can be exacerbated by stress or erratic eating habits. Some powerful antibacterial foods can reduce the risk of developing them.

Foods to eat: orange (p.18); banana (p.23); broccoli (p.94); bio-yogurt (p.151); garlic (p.248); chilli (p.252)

STRESS
The effects of stress release the hormone adrenaline in the body, as well as the potentially more harmful cortisol. In excessive amounts, this can be detrimental to health. Symptoms range from anxiety and headaches, to exhaustion and other more severe complications.

Eating the right foods can calm anxiety and irritation just as they can lift depression. Pulses, for example, contain plenty of potassium for calmness and magnesium to promote relaxation.

Foods to eat: banana (p.23); apricot (p.58); avocado (p.64); asparagus (p.78); seaweed (p.134); duck (p.145); Brazil nut (p.188); flaxseed (p.192); sunflower seed and oil (p.198); barley (p.208); brown rice (p.216); soya bean (p.224); aduki bean (p.228); kidney bean (p.230); green tea (p.264); chamomile (p.267)

Index

Acknowledgements

The publishers would like
to thank Peter Jarrett at
Middlesex University for
denoting herbal samples,
and Beatriz Linhares for
providing and preparing
herbs for photography.